# sleep sense

**Dr Katharina Lederle is a** human sleep and fatigue specialist who helps people improve their sleep and live their lives to the full. Katharina gained an MSc in Biosciences at Ruprecht-Karls University, Germany. She then completed a PhD in Human Circadian Physiology & Behaviour (the human body clock) at the University of Surrey, UK. Her PhD looked at the effects of light on human sleep patterns, specifically in the elderly. Katharina is also trained in Mindfulness and Acceptance Commitment Therapy, which she uses in her work with insomnia clients. Based in London, she has worked with a number of sleep-centred organizations, including Clockwork Research where she advised national and international airlines, emergency helicopter services, petrochemical and mining companies around the world on sleep and fatigue. She also provides sleep consultancy services to a range of businesses, including The Sleep School and pharmaceutical companies. Katharina is co-founder of Somnia, an organization that raises awareness about the importance of healthy sleep and provides one-to-one sessions, sleep workshops and educational talks helping people sleep well and feel good.

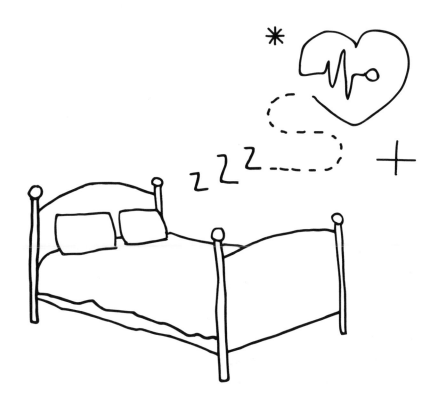

# sleep sense

## IMPROVE YOUR SLEEP, IMPROVE YOUR HEALTH

Katharina Lederle, MSc PhD

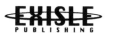

EXISLE PUBLISHING

'A book that is a pleasure to read! Clearly stated and engagingly written, Katharina Lederle draws on her research expertise and work experience to explain the latest scientific knowledge about sleep and why good sleep matters so much to our health and wellbeing. Her inviting practical approach to making sleep a priority is easy to implement in daily life — it combines science with an understanding of the reader's everyday life. A recommended read!'

— Professor Debra J. Skene, Sleep and Circadian Rhythms Researcher

'This is a very fluid read, it describes all facets of sleep in deep detail that anyone can understand. Every sleep condition is covered and it serves as a very good guide of how to improve your sleep for any reader. I found the hints throughout to be particularly useful. After reading it I realised I have bad sleep habits, and understanding the long-term effects (not evident in the short term) has made me change my habits, by prioritising my sleep.'

— Dr Justin Hamilton, Subsea Controls Engineer at BP

'I enjoyed reading both the science behind sleep alongside the practical examples everyone can relate to. I get up for an early commute every day just before 5 a.m., and hence my average sleep duration is only about 6 hours. This book has made me challenge myself rather harder as to how I can change my work/life balance somewhat to get my average weekly sleep duration closer to 7 hours (the minimum recommendation). An interesting read!'

— Will Jones, Vice President Business Operations at Fiserv FINkit

'Nothing could be more fundamental to our healthy functioning and wellbeing than sleep, and yet it can often be a focus for worry. When rest eludes us, we can over-analyze, over-medicate, and over-complicate in our search for a solution. In a straightforward, easily accessible style, *Sleep Sense* informs us about the simple building blocks of healthy sleep, and teaches us to work with, rather than against, our natural and individual sleep patterns. Her expertise makes Dr Lederle a perfect coach to help us implement the behavioural changes necessary to achieve not just better sleep, but a healthier life.'

— Dr Elaine Kasket, HCPC-Registered Counselling Psychologist

'A very helpful, practical and balanced perspective on sleep — encouraging us to look at sleep as a mindful activity to be prioritised, but also to feel relaxed about it, accepting occasional changes in sleep experience as normal rather than worrying about sticking to a rigid pattern.'

— David Champeaux, Director, Global Cognitive Health Solutions at IPsoft

### Praise for Dr Lederle

'Dr Kat has been an invaluable source of advice on sleep and the problems that we can all encounter when life takes an unexpected turn. But just as importantly, her patient and gentle approach soothes like a warm blanket in times of need.'

— Dr Stuart Greig

'I found Dr Kat incredibly helpful. Her expertise is reassuring in addition to which she's a great listener, so I came away feeling I'd been heard and had a programme designed to meet my particular needs. *I was particularly impressed by how generous* she was in replying to my emails asking for further advice and reassurance, which she was always ready to give.'

— Mark Wakefield

'After a lifetime of poor sleep, I bless the day I had my first consultation with Dr Kat. She was so supportive and encouraging — she always understood what I needed and my sleep is now improving. I never thought I'd be able to sleep well again. She has taught me so much and I will be forever in her debt.'

— Valerie

'My students were fascinated by Dr Lederle's guest sessions, the far-reaching influence that sleep has on our lives was expertly presented, and the breadth and depth of Dr Lederle's knowledge is very impressive.'

— Nigel Brown, Lecturer

First published 2018

Exisle Publishing Pty Ltd
PO Box 864, Chatswood, NSW 2057, Australia
226 High Street, Dunedin, 9016, New Zealand
www.exislepublishing.com

A CiP record for this book is available from the National Library of Australia.

ISBN 978-1-925335-73-6

Designed by Sarah Anderson
Typeset in Adobe Garamond 11.5 / 16.5
Illustrations by David Denni
Printed in China

This book uses paper sourced under ISO 14001 guidelines from well-managed forests and other controlled sources.

10 9 8 7 6 5 4 3 2 1

**Disclaimer**
This book is a general guide only and should never be a substitute for the skill, knowledge and experience of a qualified medical professional dealing with the facts, circumstances and symptoms of a particular case. The nutritional, medical and health information presented in this book is based on the research, training and professional experience of the author, and is true and complete to the best of their knowledge. However, this book is intended only as an informative guide; it is not intended to replace or countermand the advice given by the reader's personal physician. Because each person and situation is unique, the author and the publisher urge the reader to check with a qualified healthcare professional before using any procedure where there is a question as to its appropriateness. The author, publisher and their distributors are not responsible for any adverse effects or consequences resulting from the use of the information in this book. It is the responsibility of the reader to consult a physician or other qualified healthcare professional regarding their personal care. This book contains references to products that may not be available everywhere. The intent of the information provided is to be helpful; however, there is no guarantee of results associated with the information provided. Use of drug brand names is for educational purposes only and does not imply endorsement.

**To my parents
and Alexander**

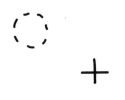

# CONTENTS

Welcome 1

Introduction 3

**Part 1: A short tour of sleep** 9

1. Sleep: the most frequent questions answered 11
2. Light and sleep 37
3. Sleep in women 53
4. Dreaming 65

**Part 2: Why healthy sleep matters** 77

5. Sleep and physical health 81
6. Sleep well to perform well 99
7. Emotional wellbeing and sleep 109

**Part 3: When sleep goes wrong** 127

8. Sleep-related breathing and movement disorders 131
9. Chronic insomnia disorder 139
10. Hypersomnias 149
11. Parasomnias 155
12. Circadian rhythm sleep–wake disorders 167

**Part 4: Weaving healthy sleep habits into your life** 177

13. A scaffolding for a healthy sleep 181
14. Dealing with sleep issues 193

Parting words 201
Glossary 203
Acknowledgements 207
References 208
Further reading 213
Index 215

# WELCOME

I'm Katharina Lederle. My clients call me Dr Kat. My dad calls me Ninchen (which means 'little Katharina'), but he's my dad so he's allowed! That aside, I'm what people refer to as a sleep specialist, therapist and educator. In other words, I help people improve their sleep and ultimately their wellbeing. The short answer to why I wrote this book on sleep, and who for, is that I want to raise awareness of sleep and how vital it is for a healthy life. By doing so I hope to have a positive impact on the lives of as many people as possible. Many more than I can reach through educational talks or one-to-one sleep therapy sessions.

There are three things I want you to take away from this reading this book. First, occasionally sleeping a little less or a little more, going to bed a little earlier or a little later than what's normal for you is just that: normal. Second, your lifestyle and behaviour can have a huge impact on the quality and quantity of your sleep. If you experience sleep problems regularly or often shift your sleep timings, then that can have negative consequences for your sleep and your quality of life. Third, by making sleep a priority — and that doesn't mean you must follow a strict routine every day — you keep your sleep healthy and yourself healthy. That in turn will benefit your family and friends, because a healthier you is a happier you.

What's not to love!

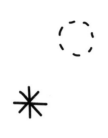
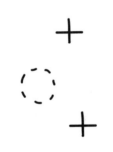

# INTRODUCTION

I've written this book to help you understand what sleep is and why it matters. It will help you gain a better understanding of the importance of sleep and the fundamental role sleep plays in your everyday life. It will help you recognize when your sleep has gone a little off-track, and will also help you get to the heart of why this might be, to take the right actions, make positive changes to sleep better and feel good as a result.

If you're a person with a busy lifestyle — maybe a working mum or dad or a busy professional — you'll learn more about how sleep affects your physical health, cognitive performance and emotional wellbeing. It will help you optimize your sleep in a way that helps boost your performance and productivity.

The sleep habits and hints this book contains give you simple and easy-to-apply insights about how to maintain a healthy, happy emotionally balanced life — *naturally*.

To make the content of this book as relevant as possible, I asked my family (including my dad — he's a farmer so he gets up early!) what their burning questions on sleep were. Some of what they came back with is answered in Chapter 1. Other questions from them, as well as from my clients, informed entire chapters such as those on sleep and health and wellbeing. One of the most frequent questions I get asked is, 'What can I do to improve my sleep?' To some extent this depends on why you don't sleep enough, so a quick answer is rarely efficient. I've included 'Part 4: Weaving healthy sleep habits into your life' where I'll discuss different strategies. Ultimately, it's about developing and implementing healthy sleep habits for yourself. But to give you the one overriding strategy right here at the start of the book: make sleep a priority in your life.

Where possible, I've included examples from friends and family members who occasionally experience poor nights. Their stories will tell you what they experienced during the evening and night, how they tried to remedy the situation, and what impact that had. My hope in sharing these personal stories is twofold: firstly, that you'll find the stories engaging and that they'll resonate with you. And secondly, that through them you'll be able to learn to quickly identify why you struggle with sleeping soundly, what skills would be most helpful in particular situations, or what you can do to minimize the occurrences of poor nights.

Did you notice that I said 'minimize' rather than 'prevent' poor nights? That's because poor nights are part of normal sleep. Sleep isn't an absolute constant. Just as you might occasionally have a bigger or smaller appetite, or get ill with a cold for a week, you might occasionally sleep a little less or a little more than what's normal for you. Sometimes you might be able to identify a particular reason, while at other times you can't. The point is that this is part of normal life, and you don't have to worry or get stressed about not sleeping 'properly' for a few nights. When your sleep is back on track, aim to get the recommended seven to nine hours, or whatever your personal sleep need is. The healthier your sleep, the more easily you can deal with sleep outliers.

There's a difference between an occasional poor night and regularly sleeping too little, though. In the next part of the introduction I'll highlight some findings from a recent international sleep survey that compared how long people said they slept with how much sleep they said they needed to function optimally. Not surprisingly, there was quite a gap between the two.

At the end of each chapter I'll give you a little summary to highlight the key points, along with suitable helpful hints throughout. It's the last section, Part 4, that I really hope will show you ways to make sleep a priority.

---

This book is for healthy sleepers, for people with an interest in sleep and those who want to learn more to optimize their sleep. An occasional poor night is part of normal sleep, part of normal life. This book is not intended as a resource for those with an ongoing or repeatedly occurring sleep problem. If your sleep problems persist and start to affect your daily life and wellbeing, or if you suffer from chronic insomnia, please see your GP or sleep specialist and get checked for sleep disorders or other medical conditions. However, following healthy sleep habits as outlined in this book will assist any treatment plan.

---

# Setting the scene

You will have heard that sleeping too little has become a health epidemic in the western world. Sleep is vital for each of the three pillars of health and wellbeing: your physical health, your cognitive performance and your emotional wellbeing. It underpins all three of them. If we don't get the amount or quality of sleep we need, we run the risk of physical and mental illness.

There's a plethora of reasons we might not sleep enough, and I'll leave that discussion for the last chapter where we look at healthy sleep habits. For now, I want to share some of the findings from an international sleep survey of six western countries including the United Kingdom, the United States and Germany, to provide you with some insight into the extent of this new health epidemic. (For the entire survey report, please see p. 214.)

For the three countries mentioned, over 50 per cent of people said they get half an hour less sleep each night than they need. That adds up to quite a bit over the course of a week. Just over 40 per cent of people said that they get a good night's sleep every night; yet more than 50 per cent felt that inadequate sleep affects their mood and performance. So, if sleep is so important to how we feel and function, why aren't we making good sleep a priority?

Finally, when asked how often they looked online for information relating to sleep, over 60 per cent of respondents from the United Kingdom and Germany said they didn't look online for sleep-related information. Nearly 70 per cent of respondents from the United States did search online, but they did so rather infrequently, less than every three weeks.

This brings me back to the purpose of writing this book: to raise awareness about sleep and provide sleep education to a wider audience. I want to ignite some fascination with sleep as a topic *and* an activity! And I hope that reading this old-school book can help you to find ways to optimize and maintain healthy, normal sleep.

Enjoy the read,
Katharina

# part 1

# A SHORT TOUR OF SLEEP

Sleep is the most exquisite invention.

Heinrich Heine, 1856

# 1.

# SLEEP: THE MOST FREQUENT QUESTIONS ANSWERED

When people hear I'm a sleep specialist, they ask me all sorts of questions about sleep: what is its role and function, what regulates it and how much sleep do we need? The best way to address these questions is to give you an understanding of what normal sleep is.

I'm going to take you on a sleep tour. Along the way we'll stop off at some of the most interesting questions people ask, to give you a good overview of the topic. I'll talk about what sleep is and how it comes about. I'll explain what happens in your brain when you sleep. And why, for example, you feel sleepy after lunch. I hope to surprise you with some interesting facts and amuse you with some theories on what might help you sleep better. But above all, I hope that reading this chapter will interest you enough to want to learn more about sleep, because I see this short sleep tour as the introduction to sleep on which all the other chapters of the book build. To get the most from this book, read this chapter first and stay on the guided tour — that way you won't miss anything.

# What is sleep and why do we do it?

Sleep is a naturally occurring state that alternates with being awake. Typically, we spend one-third of the 24-hour day asleep and two-thirds awake, fully conscious of what's going on around us. Sleep is a shift in consciousness. It's a time when we 'switch off' from the world around us and become less responsive to it. However, that doesn't mean our brain and body are doing nothing while we sleep.

During sleep many diverse physiological changes take place. The purpose of sleep isn't yet fully understood; it has been hypothesized that, among other things, sleep allows both our brain and body to replenish and restore, as well as consolidating memory and strengthening the immune system. Lack of sleep, by contrast, has detrimental effects on many areas such as our physical health, cognitive abilities like memory and alertness, and emotional wellbeing.

# What makes sleep happen?

Sleep happens when specific areas of our brain simultaneously activate and deactivate. Depending on which area is activated, either wakefulness or sleep will be promoted.

The *arousal system* is responsible for keeping us awake. This system is located within the brain and consists of certain parts of the hypothalamus, basal forebrain and brainstem. The *sleep-promoting system* also sits in the hypothalamus, which is involved in controlling many physiological factors and functions in your body. Using specific neurotransmitters (messenger molecules in the brain) and a mechanism not dissimilar to an electronic on–off switch (for which the scientific term is 'flip-flop switch'), both systems inhibit one another. So if, for example, the arousal system is active it supresses the sleep-promoting system. That's what makes sleep and wakefulness mutually exclusive: you're either asleep or awake, and the switch between the two states is normally rapid and complete. However, a malfunctioning switch, where the transitions are no longer swift and wakefulness spills over into sleep or vice versa, can be a cause for sleep disorders.

Neurotransmitters are used by the brain for cell-to-cell communication. Their interactions link different brain areas to form networks which they then either activate or deactivate. Important excitatory neurotransmitters used by the arousal system include acetylcholine, orexin, serotonin and histamine (which explains why antihistamine tablets can make you drowsy), while those used by the sleep-promoting group include GABA and galanin.

Histamine, for example, makes you more alert, helps you to think more clearly and gets you motivated. GABA is the brain's major inhibiting neurotransmitter. It basically blocks the effects of the excitatory neurotransmitters. So, sleep is of the brain and by the brain. But sleep isn't just crucial for brain functioning, it's also necessary for our body and mind to function optimally.

## How is sleep regulated?

Many of us see sleep and falling asleep like flipping a light switch: if I do this and don't do that, I'll sleep. But it's not that straightforward. The cycle of being asleep and being awake is complex and involves several brain areas and signalling systems. Fundamentally, it's the interaction of two somewhat opposing processes that regulate these brain regions and signals and that regulate our sleep–wake behaviour.

One process monitors time awake and is responsible for the pressure we feel to sleep. We call this the *sleep drive* or sleep pressure. The second process is called the *circadian pacemaker* or internal body clock. This generates signals for sleep timing. It may appear a little complicated but a slow walk through the processes and a diagram can help. Take a look at Figure 1 and then let's find out what each of the two processes actually are.

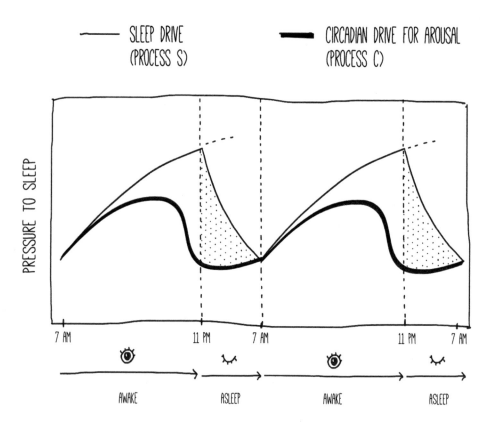

Figure 1: The interaction of the sleep and circadian drives

## The sleep drive

The sleep drive, or the need to sleep (the thin black line in Figure 1), is affected by how long you have been awake: the longer this is, the greater the pressure to sleep. The sleep drive is often likened to an hourglass, where sand flows from one side to the other (from wakefulness to sleep), and when it is full it is flipped over and the sand flows back (from sleep to wakefulness).

To explain it in detail, the longer we're awake, the more adenosine (a nucleoside) accumulates in our brain. Adenosine is a by-product of the brain's metabolic processes and is seen as a biomarker of sleepiness because it binds specific groups of cells in the brain, slowing down their activity, which makes us feel tired. The more adenosine that is bound, the greater the increase in the drive to sleep. Once levels of bound adenosine hit a certain threshold — i.e. once one side of the hourglass is full — the likelihood of falling asleep is high. That's when we feel really tired and generally go to bed and sleep. While we're asleep, adenosine disconnects and the drive to sleep dissipates — the hourglass sand flows in the opposite direction.

In typical sleepers it takes about sixteen hours for adenosine levels to reach the necessary threshold, followed by an eight-hour sleep duration. But it only takes a few hours for the drive to sleep to dissipate. So if we were to wake up at this point, after approximately four hours' sleep, we would have slept too little and this would have detrimental effects on our wellbeing and performance. Luckily the second mechanism, the circadian pacemaker, comes into play at this point.

## The circadian pacemaker

The internal circadian clock (from the Latin *circa* meaning around, and *dies* meaning day) or internal body clock acts as our body's timekeeping system. It's responsible for setting the rhythm (timing and duration) of our behavioural, psychological and physiological functions and processes, one of them being the rhythm of sleep and wakefulness.

The circadian clock comprises a specific group of neurons called the suprachiasmatic nuclei (SCN), which sit in yet another area of the hypothalamus. I like to compare the SCN to the conductor of an orchestra, setting the rhythm for the rest of the body. This is important because each organ, and in fact most of our cells, has its own clock and would function according to its own rhythm if it wasn't for the internal clock. Just as every musician in an orchestra has his or her own rhythm, without a conductor they soon would play out of time. For our bodies, the equivalent is that all our behavioural, physiological and psychological processes would be misaligned with one another as well as with the external day. We simply wouldn't be able to function in a way appropriate to the time of day if it wasn't for the master clock and its synchronizing abilities.

The internal clock has its own rhythm, which is slightly longer than the external 24-hour light/dark cycle; on average, it's around 24 hours and eleven minutes. Over time this means our internal clock will start to lag behind the external day. When this happens, our individual activities and biological processes will be mistimed or get out of sync with the external day. As a result, we exhibit the 'wrong' behaviour for a given time of day and this can have the effect of reducing our chances of good health — and survival.

To better illustrate my point, here's a short metaphor. Let's go back in human evolution and imagine it's several thousand years ago. You sleep during the day and you're awake at night, which is when you leave the safety of your cave to go hunting. Unfortunately, your night vision isn't great, so you don't notice the lioness until your head is in her mouth … her night vision is far superior to yours.

Obviously, this isn't an ideal state to be in. To prevent this from occurring, the clock needs to be synchronized by environmental time cues (known as *zeitgeber*, German for 'time giver') on a daily basis to be aligned with the solar 24-hour day. The 24-hour light/dark cycle is the strongest of these time cues; 'lights on' signals daytime and 'lights off' signals night-time to the clock. Your internal clock then relays this information via the hormone melatonin to the rest of your body. (In Chapter 2 I'll come back to this and explain how light impacts your internal clock and how it regulates the production of melatonin.)

The key point here is that your internal clock regulates when to sleep — and when not to sleep — during the 24-hour day. It maintains a separation of wakefulness and sleep, dividing them into different episodes with one during the day and the other at night, and perhaps a short one in the afternoon.

## How does this help us to stay asleep?

How do the need to sleep and the internal clock interact?

In the early morning hours, when the sleep drive has dissipated and the 'sleep' side of the hourglass is empty, arousal from sleep becomes much more likely. At the same time, the circadian clock sends out a sleep-promoting signal to consolidate our sleep and prevent us from waking up too early. Once this signal ends, we wake up and the 'sleep' side of the hourglass starts to fill up again over the course of the day.

## Is there such a thing as deep sleep?

Yes, there is. And there are even a number of other sleep stages, too. First of all, the brain shows distinct waves during wakefulness *and* sleep. Using polysomnography, where electrodes are attached to your head, researchers can record brain waves.

Sleep itself can further be divided into two broad states: rapid eye movement sleep (REM), characterized by fast, wake-like waves, and a quieter, non-rapid eye movement sleep (NREM). The repetition of alternate NREM and REM stages results in sleep cycles, each with a duration of 90 to 120 minutes. For the typical sleeper, this equates to four or five cycles per night. The graphical representation of this sleep-stage cycling is called a *hypnogram* — it's the line that goes down and up in Figure 2 (I'm a great fan of visualizing things during a discussion). When I explain a hypnogram I often compare sleep to a symphony and the hypnogram to the score.

The squiggly lines on the left are the brain waves for each sleep stage. NREM sleep can be subdivided into three stages, each reflecting a different depth of sleep.

### NREM stage 1

We enter sleep via NREM stage 1 (N1). This is a very light sleep: you become drowsy, your eyes move slowly and your muscles start to relax. Your brain waves also start to slow down and their oscillations become bigger — we call them theta waves. This is a transitional phase from

# HYPNOGRAM

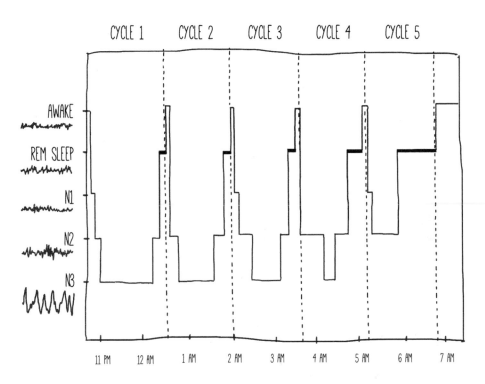

Figure 2: The hypnogram

wakefulness to sleep, when you're neither fully here nor there, you're simply gently drifting off to sleep. For example, if your partner says your name while you're in this phase you're likely to respond, and you can still detect certain types of smells. You may also experience sudden twitches or muscle spasms, called hypnic myoclonic or hypnic jerks. These are nothing to worry about. They're just an involuntary twitch of a muscle — *hypnic* is short for *hypnagogic*, meaning that it's happening during the transition from wake to sleep.

Since N1 is a lighter stage of sleep we can often misperceive such sleeping for being awake. For those lucky enough to have a bedfellow, have you ever turned to your partner to say, 'I didn't sleep last night' only to have your partner look at you and say, 'Yes, you did'? It may have been that during that night your sleep was disturbed and you spent more time in N1 than usual and you interpreted your feeling of unrefreshed sleep as a lack of sleep altogether. However, if such feelings occur regularly then it's important to see a sleep specialist to check for any potential sleep disorder, such as insomnia.

## NREM stages 2 and 3

NREM stage 2 (N2) sleep is also a light phase of sleep, though one during which everything's taken down a notch. It becomes more difficult to be woken up from N2 compared to N1. We see rapid brain wave features called sleep spindles and K-complexes appear in addition to more of the theta waves I've already mentioned. And on a physiological level, we observe a decrease in body temperature and a slowing down of breathing and heart rate.

NREM stage 3 (N3) is what is called Slow Wave Sleep (SWS) or 'deep sleep'. The dominating brain waves we see now are slow, big delta waves, and the amount of SWS correlates to our sleep drive or pressure, meaning that the higher the pressure (for example, because we have gone to bed later than the usual time), the more SWS will occur during the following sleep period. It takes some effort to wake someone up out of deep sleep; breathing, heart rate and blood pressure slow down even more and the body temperature drops further. The muscles are even more relaxed, but are still active. N3 is the phase of restoration and it helps the consolidation of fact-based memories such as learning new vocabulary for your German class or events you have experienced that day, for example. (By the way, sleep spindles also occur in N3 and might play an important role in memory formation and learning, too.)

## REM sleep

Finally, we come to REM sleep, which gets its name from rapid, rolling, eye movements. In fact, your eye muscles are the only muscles you can use during this stage. The rest of your body is almost paralysed. There might be some occasional twitches in the peripheral muscles, but for most muscle groups we experience atonia to protect ourselves from acting out the often vivid dreams that can happen during REM sleep. (Incidentally, we also dream in NREM, but our dreams are more thought-like, less vivid and less well remembered than those during REM sleep.)

During REM sleep, breathing rate, blood pressure and heart rate are elevated compared to NREM — in fact, they're more like those of someone who's awake. If you look closely at Figure 2 you may notice that the pattern of the brain waves during REM sleep is a very active one and looks very similar to being awake. That's why this stage is also called 'paradoxical sleep'. REM sleep is often linked to the consolidation of motor and perceptual skills (it's about *how* to do something like riding a bike for example) but also emotional memories, since brain regions involved in emotional processing such as the amygdala and hippocampus show an increased activity during REM sleep.

– – – – – –

So, to summarize, a healthy sleeper …
+ enters sleep through N1
+ has several (four to six) sleep cycles
+ has more NREM sleep in the first third of the night
+ has more REM sleep in the last third of the night
+ spends around 75 per cent of sleep time in NREM (divided broadly as follows: N1 about 5 per cent of total sleep time, N2 about 50 per cent and N3 about 20 per cent)
+ spends around 25 per cent of total sleep time in REM.

It's also worth noting that wakefulness during the night is part of healthy sleep behaviour (5 per cent), which we'll come to in a moment.

Are certain sleep stages more critical for our health and wellbeing than others? No, not at all. While the different sleep stages enable different processes, none is more important than the others.

I said that I see sleep as a symphony. A symphony is more complex than a pop song: it has different themes that are repeated several times in a modified form as the whole piece develops. Each theme is beautiful in its own right but it's only after we've heard the entire piece, theme after theme, modification after modification, that we can appreciate the symphony in all its brilliance.

Your brain plays a specific melody each night when you sleep and the different sleep stages are the different themes. Just like in a symphony, we need each and every repeat of the sleep stages, and we need them to occur in the right proportions to each other. The hypnogram in Figure 2 (the symphony score, if you like) shows the typical sleep architecture of a normal sleeper, which has a specific polarity: the first third of the sleep period is SWS-rich with relatively little REM sleep, whereas the last third of our sleep is characterized by a preponderance of REM sleep.

## When is the best time to sleep?

In an ideal world — ideal from a chronobiologist's point of view — you sleep when your internal clock tells you to. Bedtime is when you naturally feel tired, and wake-up time is when you naturally wake up and feel refreshed. If you follow your circadian clock, then these times should be around the same time every night or day. What's important to realize is that there's no *one* bedtime that's best for all of us. (I am using bedtime and sleep to mean the same here, but for some people there might be a big gap between their bedtime and the time when they eventually turn off the light and go to sleep.) Equally, there isn't *one* wake-up time that suits all of us. Instead, people differ in their sleep timings and these variations are reflected in the common terms 'larks' and 'owls' used to describe the tendency for an early or later sleep pattern. As you can imagine, different combinations of bedtimes and wake-up times are possible. For example, you can go to bed early and wake up early, or go to bed early and wake up late. So, perhaps see larks and owls as the two opposite ends of a continuous spectrum of timing types. This is what the term chronotype (*chronos* = time) refers to, and what chronotype you are depends to some degree on your genes, age and gender.

Sleeping according to your personal internal clock has real health benefits. It helps keep all other behavioural, psychological and physiological processes in your body in sync with each other. If you eat very late at night, it will take your body quite some time to digest the meal because the stomach isn't prepared to deal with food at this time. Usually you would be asleep and food would only arrive in the morning, so it isn't expecting any. As a result, your sleep–wake rhythm and eating rhythm become misaligned and if you continue to live against your internal clock this can lead to serious physical and mental health problems.

## How can you find out what your individual sleep timings are?

You could do the following: take five days' holiday (or longer if possible), stay at home, and go to bed and wake up as and when your body tells you to. This way you're simply following your body's natural rhythm rather than external demands. It's important to not drink alcohol or use any devices such as your tablet or smart phone too close to bedtime, as these activities will impact your natural sleep–wake rhythm — which is what we want to find out about. It's likely that your body will use the first three or four days to recover from any sleep debt you have accrued in the past. After the fourth or fifth night, you'll know *when* you sleep best.

Once you've figured out your personal sleep timings, try to stick to them — keep your sleep times as regular as you can. By that I don't mean you can't have a late night or a lie-in on the weekend. But the more regular the rhythm, the more robust and able to bounce back the clock is. For a weekend lie-in, an extra half an hour or so is fine, but then get up.

Another way to find out which chronotype you are is to complete a questionnaire such as the Munich Chronotype Questionnaire. The questionnaire asks you about your sleep timings on work days and free days. Based on what's called the midpoint of your sleep, it establishes your chronotype. (For more on the Munich Chronotype Questionnaire, see 'Further reading', p. 213.) Observing your mood in the morning might also give you some indication of your chronotype. (Have you ever looked across the breakfast table at your partner and thought, 'Please slow down!'? If this scenario sounds familiar, you could be towards the later end of the spectrum between early-larks and late-owls.)

I have already briefly mentioned why it is so critical to sleep according to your internal clock setting and to stick with it (at least on most nights), but there is another very important reason why you need to know your internal preference for sleeping. I have spoken to many people who think they have to be asleep by 11 p.m. and out of bed no later than 7 a.m. When I ask why, they say something like, 'Well, isn't the best sleep before midnight? I've also read that we all need 8 hours of sleep, so I try and get them … but it is quite hard because I don't feel tired at 11 p.m.' What is this belief based on? I am not sure, but my guess is that the many proverbs have a role to play in the origin of this belief, with their emphasis on the importance of going to bed early and rising early, with the thinking that otherwise you are lazy. But this can then lead to worrying about not sleeping, which in turn can cause a real sleep problem!

- - - - - - - - - - - - - - - - - - - - - - - -

When we sleep is highly individual and depends on several factors including genes, age and sex, as you'll see in a later chapter. While there's some change during our life, a temporal preference is always there. Given our body clock needs to be kept in sync with the solar 24-hour light/dark cycle, we need to keep our bedtime and wake-up time as regular as possible. If we don't, the clock gets confused and we may suffer consequences such as lower performance and even increased risk of disease.

- - - - - - - - - - - - - - - - - - - - - - - - -

## How much sleep do I need?

The amount of sleep each of us needs varies from person to person. It depends to some extent on our genes, our age and when we sleep. Similar to the sleep timings it's important to know what your sleep need is. It's important not to beat yourself up for what you may think is too little sleep compared to others, or that you don't increase the risk of developing health issues due to an actual lack of sleep (which, sadly, is more likely to be the case these days).

Many people believe they need eight hours simply because that is what they read and hear about. While this amount might be in the right ballpark for the majority of people, it doesn't apply to every one of us. As I said before, age and genes play a role and, perhaps, to some degree the season of the year when determining someone's sleep duration. In fact, the range is quite large when it comes to how long people need to sleep to feel refreshed in the morning. About 60 per cent of the adult population need approximately 7 to 9 hours, and while any duration between 6 and 10 hours can be appropriate, I would probably need to ask a few more questions to form an opinion on what is right for a particular individual. In 2015 the National Sleep Foundation (NSF), an independent non-profit organization which is the global voice of sleep health, published recommendations for sleep durations (see Figure 3) for different age groups, thus acknowledging the fact that the amount of sleep one needs changes throughout life. Children need more sleep while older people need less. I want to emphasize that these are *guidelines* rather than strict rules — you might need more or less, but you may also be getting the right amount for you.

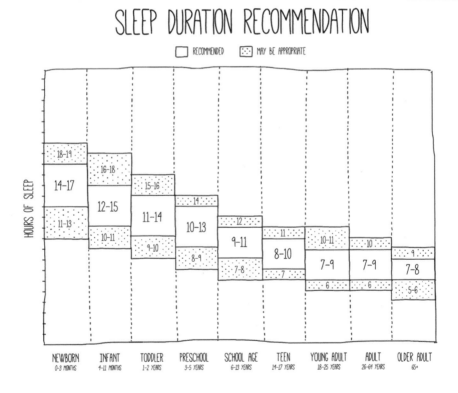

Figure 3: Sleep duration as recommended by age

The NSF included a column called 'May be appropriate', which reflects this variation in sleep durations between people. Apart from age, gender can determine how much sleep people need, with women needing a bit more sleep than men. We will look at women and sleep more closely in Chapter 3.

Your sleep behaviour changes as you go through life. Neither the amount of sleep needed and the different sleep stages, nor the timing of your sleep stays the same. The younger you are, the more sleep you need. Later in life your sleep need naturally declines, mainly due to changes in your internal clock but other health conditions may also play a part. This biological decline is reflected in the NSF's recommendations on sleep duration.

Changes in sleep architecture become most noticeable from your forties onwards. Your sleep becomes a bit lighter and more fragmented and so you tend to wake up more during the night. But these night-time awakenings might also be a result of having to use the bathroom, health issues including sleep disorders and an inability of the internal body clock to promote continuous sleep. Another reason affecting women is the menopause (see Chapter 3). Reductions in REM sleep start to occur later in life after the age of 50.

Our sleep pattern also changes, and as we grow older sleep timings shift back and forth. Young children are typically early chronotypes but become later chronotypes throughout adolescence. It isn't that teenagers don't want to go to bed, they simply can't because their internal body clock is delayed. Unfortunately, the use of electronic devices in the evening and late at night doesn't help, so there might be an element of 'not wanting to'. From around the age of 19 for women and 20 for men, the timings shift and we become 'earlier' again.

I think it's important to know that changes are likely to happen, and to have realistic expectations for your age rather than worrying too much when you notice a change in your sleep. What it comes down to is how you feel during the day — do you feel refreshed and in a good mood most days, or do you lack energy and feel low? If so, go and see your GP or sleep specialist. It might also help to review your current lifestyle and the nature of your job, as both can affect your sleep (think of them as superimposing over your biological factors).

What ultimately matters is that you know what *your* personal sleep need is. One way to find this out is to do the same experiment I suggested earlier for finding your sleep times: take those five days away from your usual commitments and sleep when and how long you like. By discovering your natural sleep–wake rhythm you automatically find the times you sleep best and how much sleep you need to wake up feeling refreshed in the morning.

You might discover that you need a lot more sleep than you realized. Many people tell themselves that they get by on six hours of sleep, thinking: 'Maybe I'm a bit tired during the day, but I can still function.' Doing this little experiment and getting the amount of sleep you actually need may leave you feeling more energized and refreshed in the morning.

I don't want you to become overly obsessed with 'achieving' your sleep need every night — just try to allow for it most nights. As we saw with the sleep timing, the more often you keep to your sleep need the easier it is for the system to deal with a night of less sleep. You should also remember that we're humans and not machines — sometimes you might sleep less than usual. This could be due to having a cold, to noise or for no apparent reason. Unless this spell of poor sleep continues for longer than two weeks, there's no need to be concerned. Just don't change your habits; it's the change in habits that could make things worse.

Do you always eat the same amount at exactly the same time every day? Probably not. You may have in mind an amount of food you consider normal for you to eat, but there'll be days when it varies; for example, a special occasion where you eat more than usual, or you get a cold and it affects your appetite. Does that worry you? Most likely not. In a way, it's the same with our sleep, some nights you may sleep less than usual and there'll be nights when you remember more of those nocturnal awakenings. And that's fine. Good sleep can vary. The key is not to get stressed about this — life isn't exactly the same every day, is it?

## Sleep debt

You might be thinking, 'What if I've missed out on a couple of hours during the week because I had a parent evening at school and a work function the next evening? Can I make up for my lost sleep?' Yes, you can. Again, researchers have come up with a name for this lost sleep: *sleep debt*.

Sleep debt is similar to a financial debt, apart from the payback mechanism. You don't have to pay back a sleep debt hour-by-hour. Just go to bed a bit earlier the next night (or nights), perhaps half an hour or so, but not much more. Otherwise you'll confuse your clock and things will get out of whack even more. You can also have a sleep-in in the morning, but my guess would be that if it's not a weekend then that won't be possible. The same goes for a nap. If you can, take a 30-minute nap the next day (but no later than 3 p.m. — the reason for this will be covered in more detail in Part 4).

Now, while it's possible to pay back some sleep debt, such as what might be incurred from a night of no sleep or one or two nights of short sleep, chronic sleep loss is much harder to pay back, if at all. Like with a bank, you can borrow money and pay it back but that comes at a cost and the bank will keep a record of your borrowing. For the body and brain this means that your health and wellbeing might become affected by long-term sleep loss. To help combat chronic sleep loss, see Part 4, 'Weaving healthy sleep habits into your life'.

## HELPFUL HINT

Importantly, chronotype and sleep duration are two fundamental aspects of sleep but they aren't dependent on one another. Whether you've a preference to get up early or later has nothing to do with the amount of sleep you need. There are early birds who are long sleepers and owl-types who need less sleep. As long as you follow your internal clock and feel refreshed then there's nothing to worry about.

## Why do I wake up during the night?

Remember the sleep stages and that we sleep in cycles? As we discussed earlier, depending on what sleep stage we're in, noise or other environment-related things can wake us up. However, we naturally wake up several times during the night, mainly at the end of each sleep cycle when we're transitioning from REM sleep to N2 sleep (N1 sleep mainly occurs at the start of the very first sleep cycle; it's the transition from wakefulness to sleep). Usually these awakenings are so brief we don't remember them and we just shift position in the bed. (Obviously, though, you're likely to remember if you get up to go to the toilet.) It's believed that these awakenings have evolved to allow us to check our environment for danger — something could be out there getting ready to eat us. Waking during the night is only a problem if you wake and struggle to get back to sleep and then feel unrefreshed the next day. If this is due to ruminating or worrying, then see Chapter 14, 'Dealing with sleep issues'.

## Why do I feel groggy when I wake up in the morning?

The answer to this question is further proof that sleep researchers and chronobiologists love giving technical names to things they observe. Process W, or sleep inertia, is what they call the grogginess most of us experience after waking in the morning. Sleep inertia is basically a state of low arousal, causing impairment of the psychological rhythms, namely your alertness and mood. What might be happening on a neural-system level is that the transition from sleep to wakefulness isn't rapid and the boundaries between the two states are fluid and overlapping: one area of the brain might be awake while another might still be asleep, so the tendency to sleep continues despite awakening.

The duration of this grogginess can be hugely different for each of us (the scientific term for this is *inter-individual* differences), and it can last from one minute to up to four hours. The length tends to depend on your genes, chronotype and how much sleep you had on the previous night/s. Once it has passed, your alertness level increases quite quickly before it then begins to settle.

Incidentally, sleep inertia is another reason why it's recommended that you keep your afternoon nap to 30 minutes or less. If you sleep longer, you're likely to enter into deep sleep (stage N3). Not only is it harder to wake up out of N3, it also takes you longer to make sense of the world around you. But if you only sleep for 30 minutes or so then you'll stay in the lighter sleep stages and come round relatively quickly.

## Eating my lunch always makes me sleepy, but why?

This is probably one of the most persistent myths about sleep. It's so persistent that many different names for this phenomenon have evolved. Scientifically known as the 'postprandial dip' (prandial relates to lunch) or post-lunch dip, it's a spike in sleepiness levels and causes a drop in alertness in the afternoon. As a result, our performance becomes temporarily impaired. Because of how close this occurs to eating lunch, the general opinion is that it must be caused by the food we eat for lunch. But have you ever noticed a spike in sleepiness levels after eating breakfast or dinner? If the rise in sleepiness is to do with eating food then why doesn't it happen in the morning or evening? At this point I need you to come on another short science excursion with me …

When we discussed the internal clock, we saw that it regulates many, if not all, processes in the body, including the rhythms of alertness, cognition and sleepiness — none of which is constant across the 24-hour cycle. The daily pattern of alertness is shown in

Figure 4. I want to take a moment to describe it in more detail. There are two peaks in alertness: one in the morning that starts after waking up, once sleep inertia has dissipated; and another in the evening as part of the wake-maintenance zone. Then there are two dips: a big one at night around 2 a.m. to 4 a.m. and another smaller dip in the afternoon, sometime around 2 p.m. to 4 p.m. — usually just after we've eaten our lunch. So rather than the post-lunch dip being caused by what you eat (although what you eat can make it worse) it's actually your internal clock that's responsible for this dip in alertness and the simultaneous spike in sleepiness.

## RHYTHM OF ALERTNESS

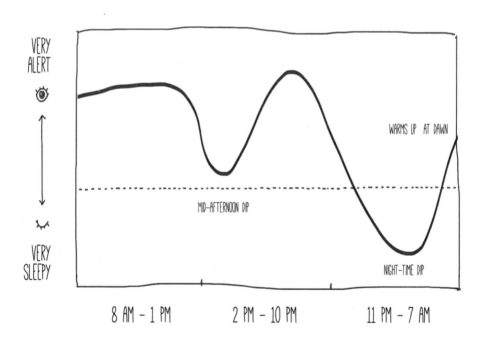

Figure 4: The daily rhythm of alertness

Why do we experience this afternoon dip in alertness? Originally it may have developed in response to the midday heat in the African savannah where humans are believed to have first evolved. Think of the siesta time in warmer climates — taking a mid-afternoon nap gets us out of the sun and heat for a while. And if we look at other species we see a similar behaviour to get through the hottest part of the day.

## HELPFUL HINT

The increase in sleepiness we experience in the afternoon is independent of eating lunch. Instead, it is a feature of the circadian rhythm of alertness (or sleepiness, for that matter) and most likely a response to the hot environment where humans first developed. Caffeine and/or a nap or walk at lunch-time can help to reduce the dip in alertness.

## Why do I get a second wind in the evening?

As weird as it may sound, this experience is a scientific phenomenon. It is because of the 'wake-maintenance zone' which is also known as the 'forbidden zone for sleep'. It has to do with a paradoxical aspect of the circadian system. While the circadian clock sends out its sleep-promoting signal during the night, quite the opposite happens during the day. Here the circadian clock sends out its wake-promoting signal to oppose the increase in need for sleep across the day.

At the end of a day, sleep pressure will reach its highest point (i.e. the 'wake' side of the hourglass is full and ready to tip over to the 'sleep' side) while in turn the circadian clock's wake-promoting signal is at its highest to prevent us from falling asleep too early. What you then experience is a sudden and very strong bout of energy a few hours before your bedtime. We are only starting to fully understand why this happens, but if we think about it in evolutionary terms, it makes sense. Historically, we would have had to have everything ready and in place before nightfall. As we can't see well at night, being out in the dark to get things organized would have put us in danger of being eaten. A sudden spike in energy levels (or 'a second wind') momentarily counteracts the increase in sleep pressure (the 'wake' side is getting fuller and fuller) and allows us to prepare and get our sleeping place ready. Interestingly, this spike in activity can also be seen in other diurnal animals (those that are active during the day).

When the wake-maintenance zone ends, we 'suddenly' feel really tired and ready for sleep. And at that point the best thing to do is to just go to bed!

# 2.

# LIGHT AND SLEEP

Lights on signals wakefulness; lights off signals sleep. That's it for a diurnal species like us. If you keep this core principle in mind it will help you optimize your sleep.

Light exerts its effect on sleep *and* wakefulness in two ways: by synchronizing your internal clock with the day, and by promoting alertness. It's important to realize that darkness mirrors these effects, telling your clock it's night-time and making you feel sleepy. Light and dark are two sides of the same coin affecting us in opposing ways.

In this chapter I'll talk about how light affects your internal clock and boosts alertness. And how that can impact your sleep by pushing the timing of it or preventing it.

But light does a little more. It also influences your mood, which I'm sure you already know from personal experience. Because the link to sleep is less direct I won't go into too much detail here other than discussing a specific form of depression called seasonal affective disorder, or SAD. For those of you who suffer from seasonal affective disorder, or know someone who does, you'll be familiar with how debilitating the daytime tiredness and change in sleeping patterns can be.

There are different parameters of light that will determine how strong light's effects on the clock and alertness will be. I'll be explaining some as we look at how light can shift your internal clock, while others will be discussed in the context of the alertness boost we experience with light.

## Light magic

Light is the strongest external time cue to align your internal body clock with the external day. This is what makes light so central to our wellbeing.

Without light, your internal clock will run according to its own rhythm, which as we have seen is longer than 24 hours for most of us. The result is a temporary, recurrent misalignment between your behaviour and psychophysiological functions on the one hand (including your sleep–wake behaviour), and the external day on the other. It's a bit like having to reset your watch every day so it doesn't lag behind the 'real' time.

Light resets or synchronizes your internal clock via a set of special photoreceptors containing a unique photopigment called melanopsin situated in your retina. Because this light-detection system is independent from our visual system it's sometimes called the non-visual system. This system has a direct connection to the internal clock in the suprachiasmatic nuclei (SCN), which it uses to transmit the light signal. When the SCN receives a 'light on' message it knows it is daytime, and when the message is 'lights off' then it knows it's night-time. The colour, pattern, intensity, timing and duration of light exposure all play a role in how light will affect our internal clock — and therefore us.

# A matter of the right colour

What I find fascinating is that within the entire spectrum of light, blue or short-wavelength light has the most powerful effect on our internal clock. We are a diurnal species and exposing ourselves to blue light or blue-enriched light during the day helps us to be awake and perform.

Exposure to blue light at night, however, is less beneficial. Its effects interfere with our sleep by misleading our internal clock into 'thinking' it's still daytime (this is called shifting the internal clock) and making us more alert. And that's where the problem lies with devices whose screen or display uses light emitting diodes (LED), such as smartphones, tablets, laptops and TVs. These devices emit a lot of blue light, so if we use them after sunset it makes sleep harder to come by and/or disturbs sleep later during the night.

A recent study by a group at Harvard University led by Anne-Marie Chang found that reading a tablet device compared to reading a book shifted the timing of the internal body clock to a later time. The internal clock sent out the 'sleepiness signal' to the body later than normal, delaying processes involved in getting us to sleep and altering sleep itself. This resulted in lower subjective sleepiness ratings before bedtime, delayed falling asleep, and a reduction in the amount of REM sleep. It also made participants more tired the next morning. All of this has implications for our daytime performance, mood, and health and safety (we'll come back to this in the chapters on general health and wellbeing).

## Regularity is key

Another important factor is the pattern of our exposure to light (i.e. how regular it is). An irregular light exposure pattern is quite naturally linked to irregular bed- and wake times. If you frequently change the time when you 'see' light, you will throw your internal clock out of whack, making it harder for it to 'predict' or anticipate upcoming demands of the external world. It will also struggle to know which internal processes need to be initiated to meet these demands. (Remember, the one thing the internal clock really loves is routine.) An example of how our internal clock relies on regular exposure to light is the anticipation of dawn. If you regularly get up around the same time, the internal clock will expect the lights to come on at a certain time and will trigger the release of hormones such as cortisol in advance of you consciously waking up. That way you're prepared and ready to go as soon as you open your eyes.

People with no light perception often show a free-running circadian rhythm because their internal clock doesn't receive any light information and can't align itself with the external world. This means that their sleep–wake cycle, the rhythms of performance and mood, are all desynchronized from the external 24-hour day for several periods across the year. Up to 70 per cent of blind people experience this desynchronization and are thus likely to suffer from sleep problems. For some blind, and some sighted people for that matter, 'non-photic' or social cues such as mealtimes, work-times or exercise can have some influence on the clock. But for the majority of us, these aren't strong enough to keep our internal clock fully entrained.

## Heralding night-time: melatonin, the internal clock's main messenger

So, what's this sleepiness signal I mentioned earlier? I'm talking about melatonin, a hormone produced by the pineal gland of the brain. Sometimes it's called the 'hormone of darkness', a reference to its main function of signalling darkness to the body.

What's crucial to know is that light regulates the production of melatonin via your internal clock. When ambient light levels start to decrease in the evening, the internal clock uses this as a signal to trigger the pineal gland to start secreting melatonin. This secretion peaks during the night around 3 a.m. The rise in the levels of (sun) light in the morning end melatonin secretion and daytime levels of this hormone are usually very low or even absent.

Relevant to our modern-day living is the fact that the room light and especially the blue-enriched light we expose ourselves to in the evening will drastically reduce the production of melatonin. This in turn increases the time it takes us to get to sleep (or back to sleep). There are two reasons why this might happen. Firstly, melatonin makes us sleepier and helps our body temperature to cool down in the evening. Interestingly, alertness increases when melatonin is suppressed by light in the evening. So far, no causality has been established as to whether the suppression of melatonin is directly responsible for the improved alertness, but there is certainly an association between the two. Secondly, melatonin provides feedback to the internal clock and can shift the clock and its rhythm. For instance, if the onset of the melatonin signal is delayed this will further delay the internal clock itself. Melatonin's ability to affect the clock is something I'll come back to in a moment when we discuss how to minimize jet lag.

So, I've told you that melatonin is associated with an increase in sleepiness. And that is why it's believed to have sleep-promoting properties. However, there's a bit of a controversy among the scientific community as to whether it can help us with sleeping. Some people take a melatonin supplement for this reason. Factors that need to be considered are timing and dosage. I suggest that if you're considering taking melatonin to treat a sleep problem, discuss this with a sleep specialist to devise a plan that's tailored to your specific circumstances. The sleep specialist will assess at what time you start producing melatonin (called the dim light melatonin onset or DLMO). In a normal, healthy sleeper this is around two hours before their bedtime. Knowing your DLMO is critical for a successful treatment; taking melatonin up to five hours before your DLMO will advance your clock whereas taking it up to ten hours *after* DLMO will delay your clock (the next night). Think of this as pulling or pushing a ball — it either comes closer (advance) or moves further away (delay).

## When everything is lagging behind: jet lag

A quick recap: blue-wavelength light is the most powerful part of the light spectrum and the timing of light decides if and which way the internal clock shifts.

Jet lag is the term for a range of symptoms we experience when we travel across time zones. This phenomenon illustrates how a rapid change in the timing of light exposure affects your internal clock and the various behavioural and psychophysiological processes that it governs. Arriving in a new time zone usually brings with it a range of unpleasant symptoms such as nausea, feeling sleepy or alert at the 'wrong' time, finding it difficult to perform, and gastrointestinal problems. It takes the internal clock a few days to reset and synch with the timing and pattern of light that's occurring in your new location.

Most people will find it easier to adapt to westward travel compared to eastward travel. Why? When we travel west, we add hours to our day. So if, for example, you flew from Sydney to London, or from London to New York, you'd end up with an extra few hours on the day of travel. The internal clock's own rhythm is a little longer than 24 hours, so in going west our internal clock can finish the day in its own time for once — until it has reset to the new time zone.

## What can you do to minimize the symptoms of jet lag?

Devise your own jet lag travel plan. One thing to bear in mind is how the *timing* of light exposure affects the internal clock. (To me this is one of the most powerful aspects of light, considering the society we live in.) Light in the early evening will delay the clock (that is, rhythms and processes will start later) whereas light in the late night or early morning will advance the clock (so rhythms and process will start earlier). Figure 5 illustrates this.

Depending on which direction you're travelling, you can start to shift your light exposure pattern and bed- and wake-up times while you're still at home, to prepare you for your destination's new light/dark cycle. When I went to Indonesia — travelling east from Europe — I got up a little earlier on the last few days before my outward flight. As soon as I was up I went outside for 20 minutes and exposed myself to sunlight. In the evening, I did the opposite; I kept the lights dim and banned all LED screen devices. I also went to bed a little earlier than usual and although I didn't fall asleep straight away it didn't worry me. After all, I was trying to shift my clock forwards and that doesn't happen overnight. However, when I went to Brazil — travelling west — I did the opposite. I stayed up later at night, keeping the lights on. I avoided light as much as possible in the morning. My aim for this trip was to shift my internal clock backwards.

But it's not always so straightforward. If you're travelling east and crossing a large number of time zones, it might be better to aim for a delay rather than the usually advised advance. You have to consider your internal time at arrival and how this might be affected by light, too. If you arrive during your 'delay part' and are exposed to strong light, then your clock might delay instead of the desired advance. Taking melatonin in combination with a timed light exposure (or avoidance) can further help to shift the clock. But its effectiveness depends on the number of time zones crossed and when you take it.

# PHASE RESPONSE CURVE

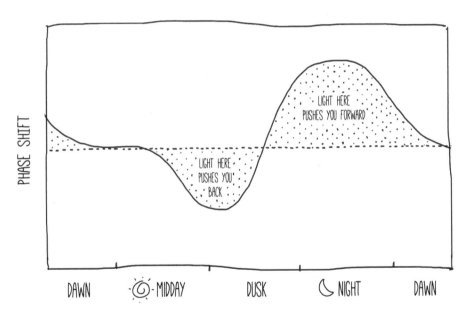

Figure 5: The phase response curve
Exposure to light in the morning (shown on the left-hand side of the figure) will make everything happen earlier, whereas light in the late evening (on the right-hand side) will make things happen later.

## Duration and intensity

What duration and intensity of light exposure is effective in assisting your internal clock and therefore your sleep? Go for as much as possible. The more time you can spend in a bright environment, the better the alignment of the internal clock with the external 24-hour day. A well-aligned internal clock will send stronger signals to the body, telling it when to be awake and when to sleep.

The same is true for alertness. Let's now look at what else there is to know about light and alertness — and sleep.

## Light enhances alertness and thus stops you sleeping

Light not only entrains your internal clock, it also acutely and directly increases your alertness and overall cognitive performance.

Melanopsin, the photopigment I mentioned earlier, picks up the light signal that enters the eyes and passes it on to the areas of the brain responsible for cognitive functioning, and light is able to improve your cognitive performance during the day and at night — up to a point. Your internal clock will naturally push your alertness during most of the day. We briefly spoke about this in Chapter 1 when we stopped off at the question about feeling tired after lunch.

In short, alertness and sleepiness are inversely related, meaning that if one goes up the other goes down. Bear this relationship in mind when reading the following paragraphs about how light affects your alertness.

You will know how stepping into the sun when you feel tired or sleepy during the afternoon immediately makes you feel more alert and able to concentrate. And the longer you spend in the bright light the more alert you feel. Similarly, waking up with a bit of light coming through the curtains or using a wake-up light can help increase your alertness in the morning, especially if you suffer from sleep inertia.

- - - - - - - - - - - - - - - - - - - - - - -

Normal indoor lighting is only 300 to 500 lux (lux being the unit of measurement of light intensity), compared to natural outdoor light, which reaches 100,000 lux on a bright sunny day. Even on an overcast day, light levels reach 1000 to 2000 lux.

- - - - - - - - - - - - - - - - - - - - - - -

And then there's the evening light exposure and the use of LED devices. The blue light emitted by your phone, tablet or laptop not only affects sleep by delaying the clock, it also makes you more alert. So, watching a movie on your tablet or reading your emails will stimulate your cognitive performance. In the study by the Harvard group I mentioned earlier, researchers also measured alertness while the participants were reading in the evening. To no one's surprise, levels of alertness were higher when reading an e-reader than when reading a book. A few nights of this won't cause a sleep problem, but if you get into the habit of reading an e-reader, or working late using your laptop or tablet, it can have a severe impact on your sleep and may add to or even start sleeping problems.

So we now know that light of high intensity and/or blue-enriched light stimulates your alertness and keeps you awake. What about the opposite?

## What about darkness and sleepiness?

Have you ever sat in a comfortable chair listening to a musical performance in low-light conditions thinking, 'I'll just close my eyes, just for a second …'? The next thing you remember is your friend giving you a nudge to wake you up. Most of you will have first-hand experience of how dim lights in the evening, such as at the movies, can make you feel sleepy. One could say that the dim light isn't strong enough to support the internal clock's signal to stay awake (see 'Why do I get a second wind in the evening?' on p. 35 in Chapter 1) and that's why you feel the effects of the sleep pressure building up. As soon as you get into a well-lit environment you perk up again, at least for a moment (a change in posture will have some effect, too).

## HELPFUL HINT

To use light as an alertness booster, consider its colour, intensity and duration. The more time you can spend in a well-lit environment, the better. There might just be one small caveat: time of day. Alertness is naturally on the rise in the morning and so might be less responsive to light.

Ideally, avoid using your LED devices altogether in the evening and switch them off for the night. Where that's not possible, install blue-light filters and aim to not use devices for one hour prior to bedtime. What's more important: that work email that could potentially shift your clock and keep your mind engaged, or your sleep health? I guess you know my answer to that.

## Effects on mood

We all know about the effects of light on our everyday mood and vitality. Being outside on a bright, sunny day (where we are exposed to light that contains short-wavelength light) or in a well-lit room instantly makes us feel better and lifts our mood. If, on the other hand, the lighting is dark, our mood declines and we can feel sluggish and low. Just think of how you feel during the early days of spring coming out of a long, dark winter. Interestingly, if the light gets too bright — perhaps too 'cool' — your mood may start to decline again.

How does this relate to sleep? It's right to be sceptical, as there's no straightforward relationship — it's not as simple as 'light lifts your mood and so you sleep better'. You might even lie in bed wide awake, excited about what life is offering. How mood and sleep influence one another is discussed in detail in Chapter 7. However, at this point I want to tell you more about seasonal affective disorder (SAD) or 'winter depression'. This affects people living in northern countries and is a good example of how light can have a profound impact on our mood.

SAD manifests itself during autumn and winter, when light levels are much lower in countries of moderate and higher latitude, such as Scandinavian countries. A low mood or feeling depressed, greater sleep need and fatigue, and overeating (especially carbohydrates) are the main symptoms of SAD. Light therapy is the recommended treatment. There is a plethora of light boxes available that differ in the spectrum (either white or blue-enriched), intensity and type of light bulb (traditional tube bulb or LED therapy device) they use. When you choose a light therapy box, ensure you buy it from a certified manufacturer, a company that has proven research in this field; that way, you know it'll be effective.

Light therapy for SAD is generally more effective when administered in the early morning hours. But optimizing the timing to suit your individual chronotype is what shows the best results in alleviating symptoms. The website for the Center for Environmental Therapeutics provides a link to an online questionnaire to help you establish your personal exposure timing. See 'Further reading', p. 213, for more details.

How SAD is caused isn't exactly clear, but a disturbance of the internal clock due to lack of light has been hypothesized to be part of the underlying mechanism/s. Individuals who suffer from SAD are often less sensitive to light, making it harder for their internal clock to tell the correct time when there is less light outdoors. This might cause a misalignment of their behavioural and psychophysiological processes and rhythms — with one another as well as the external world. As a result, sufferers sleep longer, earlier or later than what is normal. In addition to the possible misalignment, lower serotonin levels during the darker months might also play a role in affecting mood as well as the internal clock's reduced sensitivity to light.

The therapeutic effects of light exposure are not exclusive to the treatment of SAD. Other mood disorders including bipolar and unipolar depression and the symptoms of jet lag benefit from the ameliorative effects of light therapy, either as a standalone or as an adjunct treatment.

## To sum up

Light affects sleep via the internal clock, by shifting it to an earlier or later time. You can use this to prepare when travelling across time zones. Late-night exposure to blue light can delay sleep onset, potentially reducing your overall sleep time.

Light also affects sleep via its alerting effects: light during the day, and more so during the night, will stimulate your alertness and performance and reduce your sleepiness.

The timing of your exposure to light, along with its colour, pattern, intensity and duration all play a role in how light will affect you.

Most indoor light settings don't resemble the conditions we've evolved under as a species. They aren't able to affect our internal clock, alertness and mood. Natural daylight is still the most effective for keeping our internal clock aligned with the external day.

Knowing how light influences your behaviour and psychophysiology, it might be worth rethinking the lighting conditions you experience in your daily life. Can you spend more time outside during the day, particularly in the morning? Can you reduce the amount of blue light in the evening, and perhaps discuss light installations at your workplace?

# 3.

# SLEEP IN WOMEN

While sitting over our second coffee of the afternoon, my friend Abby and I stumbled onto the subject of sleep. She told me: 'I always know when I have ovulated because I feel hot and sweaty. I also feel much more tired during the day. But what annoys me the most is that my sleep gets really poor two nights before I start my period. I toss and turn and wake up a lot during the night, sometimes three times. And so the following days become a bit of a struggle, to be honest.' When I asked her what she did to manage the tiredness during the day she said, 'I drink a lot of coffee so I can still go out with George in the evening. He always has more energy than me in the evening!'

If you're a woman then it's likely that this story resonates with you to some degree. When asked to subjectively assess their sleep in surveys, women tend to report more sleep problems than men. The biggest complaint from women, apart from poor sleep quality, is the overall lack of sleep and how this affects them during the day. Other complaints include finding it difficult to fall asleep at bedtime and waking up several times during the night, and once having woken finding it hard to get back to sleep.

Interestingly, when sleep is measured using polysomnography (assessing sleep using electrodes measuring brain waves; see Chapter 1) women appear to have better sleep quality than men. There's a discrepancy between subjectively assessed sleep (using questionnaires) and objectively assessed sleep (via polysomnography) for women, a fact that's well known among scientists. (We'll explore this a little later in this chapter.)

I would like to highlight that sleep studies using polysomnography have historically tended to focus on men. Hence literature and findings relating specifically to sleep in women are somewhat limited. Within the pool of female sleep studies, the number of studies looking at differences in sleep between women on a natural cycle and women on oral contraceptives becomes even fewer. There's a real need for more studies investigating sleep in women to get a better picture of what sleep is like as well as being able to diagnose sleep problems and optimize treatment. But let's see what else we know about sleep differences between men and women, and what actually makes sleep in women unique. Unique does not mean abnormal, though. What makes sleep in women unique is that female biology is unique and this brings about its own set of problems or symptoms that affect sleep, and vice versa.

This chapter is aimed at both women *and* men — so that we all take these problems seriously.

## How does sleep differ between women and men?

A woman's internal body clock tends to run a little faster. The time it takes the clock to complete a cycle is, on average, about six minutes shorter compared to men. And for some women it's even shorter: less than 24 hours! Physiologically speaking, this means that the rhythms of alertness, body temperature and melatonin, for example, are shorter and start earlier. Most importantly, though, the timing of sleep is earlier for most of us women (compared to men), and that can have implications for the quality and duration of our sleep. On that note, women tend to need more sleep than men and have more deep sleep. But women also seem to accumulate a sleep debt much faster than men, and the effects of sleep loss on health may also be more severe than in men. Why this is the case is currently under investigation, but it certainly highlights the importance of regular sleep and wake times.

So what do having a faster ticking clock and earlier sleep timings mean for everyday life? If you go to bed and wake up when your internal clock tells you to, not much. But if you go to bed much later than your internal time, you are cutting into your sleep. Now you won't be able to make up for this lost sleep in the morning because your wake-up time is set by your internal and/or alarm clock. Your internal clock triggers the waking-up processes a little before it expects you to wake up, irrespective of how many hours you have slept. You might notice this as drifting in and out of sleep or poor-quality sleep in the last few hours. Eventually this can lead to insomnia and other sleep problems. Women are almost twice as likely to develop insomnia than men, and as women get older the risk of developing sleep problems generally increases.

## What makes sleep in women unique?

While sleep is usually fine during the first half of the cycle, many women feel more tired during the latter half of their menstrual cycle as a result of sleep disturbances. So what's driving these sleep problems?

Well, it's down to our cyclically changing ovarian hormonal milieu. Oestrogen and progesterone, and their fluctuating levels across the menstrual cycle, are the most powerful drivers behind the sleep problems many women experience. Often, sleep is made worse by experiencing menstrual symptoms such as tender breasts, headaches, bloating and changes in mood.

A woman's sleep also changes over her lifetime. Sleep problems may start in puberty when we experience the puberty-associated rise in ovarian hormones, and for many women sleep problems arise in periods when large hormonal changes take place. So let's now explore how sleep changes during the menstrual cycle, pregnancy, menopause and post-menopause.

## Is sleep affected by the menstrual cycle?

Women are more likely to report sleep disturbances the week before the start of menstruation and/or for the first few days of menstruation. (If you wonder whether this is true for you, keep a sleep log for two months to find out.) It can take us longer to fall asleep, we might wake up more often during the night and our sleep quality is generally poorer. Often, we feel more tired during the day, and for some of us our mood is low, too. What makes the experience of poor sleep much worse is experiencing premenstrual symptoms simultaneously. Maybe not surprisingly, women who suffer from severe premenstrual symptoms also tend to complain about more unpleasant dreams. By the way, at this time in our cycle, levels of progesterone and oestrogen are decreasing.

Interestingly, when measuring sleep objectively, changes in sleep become apparent a little earlier on in the menstrual cycle — just after ovulation, during what's called the luteal phase. During this phase, levels of progesterone are high, causing our body temperature to raise by about 0.4°C (0.7°F). Progesterone is also a soporific and so it makes you more tired — which is exactly what Abby and so many other women describe. Studies have also shown that there's more N2 sleep and slightly less REM sleep, but no change in the amount of deep sleep during the luteal phase. (See Chapter 1 if you want to remind yourself of what these different stages are.)

Let me come back to why there seems to be a discrepancy between subjectively reported sleep problems and what objective sleep studies have found. One explanation might be that factors unrelated to sleep (so-called 'sleep-independent' factors), like feelings and mood, affect how women perceive their sleep. Indeed, depressive symptoms and anxiety, both more common in women than men, can influence how we 'experience' and rate our sleep. This may lead to the more negative perception of sleep. (Many women experience mood swings during their menstrual cycle as part of hormonal changes, and this can be an influencing factor.) Mood disorders can also contribute to the development of insomnia. As I said earlier, women have a higher risk than men of developing insomnia. But insomnia or lack of sleep can also contribute to the development of mood swings and disorders. (Insufficient sleep temporarily impairs certain brain areas, making it harder to respond in an emotionally appropriate way.) Often it's not known 'which came first' so it's important to look at both your mood and your sleep if you experience problems with either or both.

Assessing sleep both subjectively and objectively is the best way to understand it better. Hence, I have included both methods in the following sections.

## What about sleep in women on oral contraceptives?

Unfortunately, there are only a few studies exploring the effects on sleep of oral contraceptives (commonly referred to as the pill). The results vary greatly between them so it's difficult to draw any final conclusions. These mixed results are, in part, due to the various oral contraceptives used and their different hormone levels and combinations. Overall, it seems that sleep and sleep quality are not adversely affected by the pill.

Some differences that have been observed include changes between the sleep stages (i.e. change in sleep architecture) and body temperature. The latter is due to the synthetic progesterone, whose levels don't fall as sharply in women taking the pill as in naturally cycling women. Body temperature stays elevated for longer after the final active pill, too. Given all we know, women who suffer from menstrual irregularities and related sleep problems may actually benefit from taking the pill. At the same time, it's clear that more research is needed — around 22 per cent of women in Europe and 16 per cent in the United States use oral contraceptives.

## What happens to a woman's sleep during pregnancy?

Perhaps unsurprisingly, the changing levels of our ovarian hormones during pregnancy influence sleep. While pregnant, sleep becomes lighter and more disrupted, and sleep architecture is altered. Levels of progesterone are rising and this is thought to play a role in why pregnant women feel so very tired. And then there's the pregnancy itself, with all its changes to the body and its physiology that can contribute to sleep problems.

Pregnant women report more problems with their sleep than non-pregnant women overall, but there are also differences in sleep between the different trimesters of pregnancy. While during the first trimester you sleep more and feel more tired during the day, most pregnant women report that sleep then improves a little during the second trimester. But by the third trimester, sleep problems get worse. Most women complain about not getting enough sleep and waking up frequently, not feeling properly refreshed in the morning and finding it harder to perform during the day. (Do you recognize these symptoms? Insomnia, yes. The NSF conducted a sleep survey among women and found that 64 per cent of currently pregnant women or those who had recently given birth report insomnia.) All of this has a huge impact on a woman's quality of life and mood, too.

As I've already said, sleep disturbances are often also a result of sleep-independent factors (in this case, factors related to the pregnancy itself). These may include heartburn, nausea, (back) pain, restless legs syndrome (discomfort and restlessness in the legs that can only be relieved by movement, which happens in the evening/ at night), periodic leg movements syndrome (sudden movement/ kicking of the whole leg; again, this happens in the evening/at night), breathing problems and the ever-increasing need to go to the toilet. They can all disturb a woman's sleep.

Apart from its thermogenic and soporific effects, progesterone also affects the body's smooth muscles by making them relax more. That might not sound like a problem, but it can cause snoring and breathing problems such as sleep apnoea (I will talk about this more in Chapter 8) and may make you go to the bathroom even more often. The fluctuating levels of progesterone and oestrogen can also impact mood and emotions. These are believed to be contributing factors in the development of mood swings or depression during pregnancy and after childbirth. (I find these findings regarding the role of progesterone and oestrogen fascinating as it shows how far-reaching the effects of our ovarian hormones are!)

About one-third of pregnant women experience some form of depression or anxiety during their pregnancy. This can further exacerbate sleep problems and, as we've already discussed, can have an effect on the subjective perception of sleep.

One final note on sleep during the postpartum period. After childbirth, hormone levels drop sharply; progesterone levels in particular show a sudden fall. This drop — together with the newborn's irregular sleeping pattern and all the other factors like feeding the baby, older children and the level of support you receive — are likely to affect your sleep quality and quantity, too. Not to mention your emotional state, which in turn may affect your sleep.

## Does menopause affect sleep?

Menopause marks another significant biological phase in a woman's life, just as a girl comes of age when she menstruates for the first time. During this stage, ovarian hormones fluctuate until they eventually decline. As part of the menopausal transition, women may experience problems such as difficulties functioning during the day, mood swings and, what we are most interested in, sleep disturbances. Intensity and frequency of these problems may vary between women and for a woman herself while transitioning. However, sleep changes are also part of normal ageing, too, and so some sleep problems we see during the menopause are likely to also be related to non-gender-specific processes taking place during this period in your life.

There are two specific factors which are likely to affect your sleep when you are going through the menopause. As you may have already guessed, one of them is yet another change in our ovarian hormones that impacts our sleep at this stage in life. The fluctuating and eventually declining levels of oestrogen, in particular, seem to play a major role in the worsening of sleep. But how?

Oestrogen has several effects on the brain, including areas and neurotransmitters involved in sleep regulation and thermoregulatory centres. We already know how important regularity is for our sleep and the body in general, so if the oestrogen signal becomes irregular it also becomes a weaker player within brain regulatory processes. Think of tennis doubles: if the performance of one partner starts to decline to the point where she eventually needs to be taken off the court, it becomes much more difficult for her partner to bring the game to a successful finish. And this is basically what's going on with the oestrogen signal to the brain — it becomes weaker. The results are problems with sleep and thermoregulation. Poor sleep quality is reported by 33 to 51 per cent of women in the menopausal transition period, for example. Other common sleep complaints include insomnia, extreme tiredness and struggling to cope during the day, and mood-related symptoms, to name just a few.

The second factor which I briefly mentioned earlier and which is the hallmark symptom of the menopause is hot flushes. These are episodes of flushing, intense heat (sometimes you might even sweat) followed by shivering and cold sensations. They occur several times during the night, often accompanied by palpitations. A whopping 75 per cent of women experience hot flushes during their menopausal transition. While intensity and frequency vary between and within individuals, hot flushes are likely to disturb the first half of your night-time sleep in particular. Hot flushes may cause or further exacerbate other problems such as insomnia or a low mood.

What's important to realize is that while the changes in ovarian hormone levels and the occurrence of hot flushes are definitely involved in causing sleep problems and dissatisfaction, it's how we react to them that can make them much worse. These are unpleasant experiences and no one enjoys feeling unrefreshed during the day. A natural reaction is therefore to try everything to get rid of them. But when the symptoms then don't go away, frustration and anger can grow. An alternative is to simply accept what's happening and that this is part of being a woman going through the menopause.

The sleep of postmenopausal women gets even lighter and more fragmented. The risk for developing a sleep problem is over three times higher during this stage than it is for premenopausal women. Insomnia and sleep apnoea are the most common complaints reported by postmenopausal women. In Part 4 I will summarize different behavioural therapies that can help you to improve your sleep, but the best way forward if you are concerned is to see your GP or sleep specialist for more advice.

## To sum up

A woman's sleep changes across her lifetime alongside many other things. Biological phenomena including menstruation, pregnancy and menopause are times when sleep problems are more likely to occur or become more pronounced. Changes in ovarian hormone levels, especially progesterone and oestrogen, are likely to be one reason. Changes in mood as well as physical complaints often contribute to sleep problems, too. It's a little bit more difficult to say what exactly causes sleep problems during the menopausal transition, though. Apart from hormonal changes, changes in mood, ageing, systemic diseases and medication might also contribute to the development of sleep problems. Early treatment has the best chance to be effective; please consult with your GP about your options.

# 4.

# DREAMING

What are dreams and why do we dream? People have been pondering this for millennia but still to this day we don't have the answers. That said, there are a number of things that have been firmly established.

In this chapter I'll tell you about two of the major theories regarding why we dream and how sleep stages affect dreams. There are gender differences in dreaming behaviour and I'll use those as a way of illustrating how daytime experiences affect our dreams.

## What are dreams?

Put simply, a dream is a subjective experience, a mental activity that takes place while you're sleeping. It's a state of consciousness where waking life — its concerns, thoughts and experiences — extends into sleep. But because it's not directly measurable, we need to be awake to become aware of and talk about it. In other words, we recall the dream. How well we recall it is another matter and one that makes dream research so difficult.

# Why do we dream?

To be frank, even in academic circles this hasn't yet been fully established, not reliably so anyway. A number of theories exist, and while some of these are plausible they all lack robust evidence, which, given the nature of dreams, is rather tricky to obtain. Research can only examine dreams that we remember. How well each of us remembers might differ from day to day and from person to person.

## Theories on the function of dreams

A full review of the theories of dream function goes beyond the scope of this book. But there are three theories I want to highlight in this chapter because they complement each other in supporting the notion that dreaming is for learning in very general terms.

The first theory sees dreaming as part of sleep-dependent memory consolidation. One of the functions of the sleeping brain is to reactivate and consolidate memories of the waking day. What happens is that important memories are moved from a short-term storage facility and encoded in a long-term storage facility within our brain. Here comes the interesting bit. Daytime events, or waking life experiences as some researchers prefer to say, are also reflected in our dreams. We incorporate waking life experiences into our dreams and by doing so we are — almost as a by-product — further aiding the consolidation of this specific memory (at least according to the memory consolidation theory).

The second theory assumes that dreams are an opportunity to be creative, helping us to come up with novel solutions for existing problems.

Most of the time, we dream about an event the following night and then again around seven nights later. Yet while current events are more prominent than events from the past, it does not mean that the latter are of no influence on what is bothering us at present. When we dream, past experiences combine with what is currently on our mind. Our brain plays through different scenarios and 'imagines' new strategies to solve the issues of our waking life. Viewed in this way, dreaming becomes an innate problem-solving process tool.

The last theory I want to discuss is the idea that dreaming plays a significant role in the regulation of our emotions, helping ameliorate the intensity of emotional events. If you think of how quickly our mood and emotions change during the day, we experience a lot of ups and downs. Dreaming might lessen the emotional turmoil of both positive and negative daytime emotions so that we regain an emotionally balanced state. As you'll see in Chapter 7 on emotional wellbeing, sleep helps to regulate mood in general. Dreaming might be one way this is achieved.

So dreaming might have more than just one function. Perhaps different dreams have different functions, and maybe that depends to some degree on what's preoccupying us in our current life. Alternatively, perhaps the sole function of dreaming is in the process of dreaming itself. Who knows?

## Does everyone dream?

Even if you don't remember them, everyone has dreams. What differs between those who can see and those who can't is the sensory composition of the dream. Depending on when the blindness occurred (congenitally or acquired during their lifetime), blind people have little or no visual content to their dreams but may have more impressions from other sensory modalities.

## Dreams and sleep stages

Most people think we only dream during REM sleep but we actually dream during NREM sleep, too. REM dreams are usually more vivid, bizarre and emotional, and possibly use more imagery. (To prevent us from acting out our dreams and potentially harming ourselves, our bodies are paralyzed while we are in REM stage; I will explain this in Chapter 8.) Dreams in NREM sleep are more like thoughts, more fragmented and less bizarre. We're more likely to remember REM compared to NREM dreams (80 per cent versus 50 per cent recall, respectively). And while different dream types and subtypes are associated with each of the two sleep stages, there may be some overlap, too. Nightmares and lucid dreams (dreams in which the dreamer knows she or he is dreaming and can direct the dream) fall under REM sleep dreams. Sleep onset dreams and night terrors come under NREM sleep dreams. Other dreams like post-traumatic nightmares occur in both REM and NREM sleep.

## The relationship between waking life and dreams

Dreams include daytime events. It's likely you've experienced for yourself that daytime thoughts, emotions and activities are reflected in your dreams, albeit in some bizarre or metaphorical form. Research talks about the continuity between waking life and dreams, your concerns, experiences and concepts continue in your dreams (the so-called 'continuity hypothesis'). By looking at the different aspects of our waking life more closely we can begin to see how it affects and almost extends into our dreams.

I've already mentioned the temporal factor — current daytime events are more prominent in our dreams than past events. Furthermore, activities we've spent more time on during the day occur more often in our dreams. So, for example, if you drive a lot, then this theme will be incorporated in many of your dreams. Yet it's the level of emotional involvement that ultimately determines how frequently any of these daytime activities show up in our dreams. The more emotionally intense a daytime experience, the more likely we are to dream about it. Studies have shown that social interactions such as spending time with friends or your partner feature more often in our dreams than cognitive activities such as reading, for example. I think it's worth knowing that the emotional tone (i.e. whether the emotional experience was positive or negative) doesn't influence the rate of incorporation into our dreams.

## Do women and men dream differently?

Apparently so, although the differences are small. Women describe their dreams as very vivid and meaningful, and tend to recall dreams more often, especially in situations of stress, compared to men. Dream content is another interesting aspect. While there are more similarities than not, some differences exist. Women dream more about clothing, the household and indoor scenarios. Men dream more about sex, weapons and physical aggression. How can we explain such gender differences? Before I talk about that, there's one thing I should mention: male erections during sleep. Every healthy man has several erections during the night while he's dreaming. But it's nothing to do with the content of his dreams. The body is just making sure that the penis is supplied with blood and checking that everything is still working. Women have erections, too, but this is less studied.

Let's come back to the differences in dream content between women and men. What's influencing these differences? As it turns out, there's more to it than just our gender. In addition to the three factors we've already discussed it's the type of daytime activity that will impact dream content.

Women and men share many of the same interests and fears, likes and dislikes in life. At the same time, there are also dissimilarities in their waking lives. Women tend to be more involved in family matters and housework, and are more likely to work indoors compared to men. We also spend some of our waking day thinking about what to wear and what we look like (at least, more than men), which could explain why clothing features so often in our dreams. The reason that men dream more about weapons might be explained by specific media consumption (e.g. playing violent computer games). The higher rate of sex in their dreams is likely because men tend to spend more time fantasizing about sex in their waking lives compared to women.

In summary, the reason women and men dream about different things isn't simply due to sex differences. It's more likely a result of social patterns — women and men engage in different quotidian activities which shape their dream content and personality type. In fact, we could look at any two groups who differ at least to some degree in their waking life and we would find similar results (i.e. differences in dream content). Interestingly — and quiet importantly, I think — personality traits also affect and modulate dream content and recall. In a recent study published in the *International Journal of Dream Research*, researchers Mathes and Schredl looked at how dream content relates to personality traits. They found that men reported more dreams about clothing if they scored lower levels of agreeability compared to men with high agreeableness scores. (People scoring lower on agreeableness place less value on getting along with others, and the researchers hypothesize that more disagreeable men are less conventional and want to stand out by way of how they dress.) Women with high scores of openness to experience in this study dreamed more often about clothing than women with lower openness scores. (People who are more 'open to experience' are generally curious about many things, possibly including clothing, as pointed out by the authors.)

And to give you an explanation of why women recall dreams more frequently than men: interest in dreams might be a driving factor for this difference. Frequent night-time awakenings and a lower sleep quality have been associated with a higher rate of dream recall. Women experience insomnia or insomnia-type symptoms more often than men and so this could be another contributing factor for the gender differences we see.

## Your dreams' relationship with waking life

If waking life affects dreams, what about dreams' influences on waking life? There's evidence that dreams affect our mood the following day. Maybe you've even noticed this yourself, how a dream you remembered when you woke up put you in a certain mood. What I find interesting, and hence worth knowing, is that although we seem to have more negative dreams (we recall these more often than positive ones) that doesn't mean that those dreams are more powerful in influencing our daytime mood.

Dream researchers have shown that, perhaps a little surprisingly, both the positive and negative emotions we experience during dreaming can equally influence our mood the next day. It's the *intensity* of the dream emotion that determines whether the dream will affect our daytime mood. (This is the same as what we have seen when we discussed the effects of waking life on dreams.) When we compare dreams with 'normal' levels of emotions to nightmares, we see that the latter have a much more pronounced effect on daytime mood. Nightmares are extremely negatively toned dreams, which cause the sleeper to wake up feeling upset, sad or scared. While these emotions are certainly distressing, it's also the frequency (i.e. the repeated experience) of nightmares that's responsible for their strong effect on our mood.

---

The reason for recurrent nightmares seems to be that the dream state struggles to ameliorate and regulate intense emotional experiences from our waking life. The experience, or rather the emotional part of it, is therefore not sufficiently processed and we find it hard to move on.

---

There is a long-held view that dreams boost our creativity. Research in this area is sparse but there are accounts of famous people such as Paul McCartney and Salvador Dalí taking inspiration from particular dreams. Many other non-famous people have also reported that dreaming has stimulated their mind and let them be more creative in everyday life. Some have tried new activities whereas others take a novel approach to an existing problem. (Perhaps this is a little experiment you could conduct yourself: try to recall your dreams and see if they lead you to a new idea.)

So there's a continuity between dreaming and waking life, just as seems to be the case between waking life and dreams. And in a way, you could think of the continuity hypothesis in reverse here.

# Discontinuity

The continuity hypothesis of dreaming makes a lot of sense, yet there are dreams where we find it hard to see any (literal or metaphorical) connection with our waking life. In other words, there is or seems to be a thematic discontinuity between waking life and dreams. These dreams include experiences never had by the dreamer — think of a congenitally blind person dreaming about experiences only a sighted person can have, or a person who is congenitally paraplegic dreaming about going for a run.

How can we explain these dreams? Science doesn't quite know yet. More research needs to be done to help us understand whether there's a disconnect between waking life and dreams or if every dream can be explained within the concept of continuity. Because even if there's no overt continuity between the person's dreams and their waking life, there might be an emotional continuity between daytime and dreaming.

# Common themes in dreams

With the assumption of the continuity hypothesis in mind, let's take a quick look at dream interpretation. This is by no means a straightforward process, as you might already know. What I find interesting is that although dreams are unique to our personal life, there are some common themes we share with others, especially with people from similar cultural backgrounds and with similar social patterns. Similarities in lifestyle, age and gender and thus waking experiences are a likely explanation for this. Take an older and a younger person. The older person reports more dreams including people who have passed away. The young person reports more dreams including elements related to learning or studying (such as teachers and schools). The reasons for this lie in the waking life. The older person is more likely to have experienced the loss of loved ones, while the young person would spend a large amount of their time in education. So, typical situations are incorporated into typical dreams.

Common themes include flying, trying something again and again, and running away. What do they mean? This is a topic of intense speculation, both non-scientific and scientific and, to be honest, no one really knows. It might be possible to assign metaphorical meanings to dreams and dream themes. Using this approach and adopting psychological concepts, one could say that dreams incorporating elements of chasing or running away might resemble an avoidance behaviour we're adopting in waking life. But there are a lot of questions unanswered and even more still to be asked. Working with dreams and dream content can be beneficial in helping us understand ourselves better (our motives and behaviours) and to be more creative. At the same time, I believe not every dream necessarily has a meaning. Hopefully, future research will bring more clarity on the functions of dreams.

## To sum up

Dreams are subjective experiences that occur during all stages of sleep. According to the continuity hypothesis, waking life extends into our dreams. Or, daytime events are reflected in our dreams. Dreams might help us to consolidate our memory and/or work things through, especially emotionally intense experiences. Since our waking life shapes our dream content (at least to some degree), it's not surprising that we see differences between men and women, as we do when comparing any two groups.

Research has discovered common themes in dreaming. This phenomenon is likely to be explained by the continuity hypothesis, where typical situations lead to typical dreams. There's speculation about the meaning of dreams, however. Nothing has been firmly established and it's hoped that future research will shed more light on plausible meanings of dreams. One thing that is clear, though, is that sleeping and dreaming aren't a waste of time — even if it's just to help us find a solution to a problem that's been bugging us for days, it's worth it!

# part 2

# WHY HEALTHY SLEEP MATTERS

- - - - - - - - - - - -

Sleep is that golden chain that ties
health and our bodies together.

Thomas Dekker, 1609

If we aren't sleeping properly it doesn't take much for us to fall ill, catch a cold or feel exhausted. When we're ill it's really important to get a good night's sleep. The saying 'Looks like he got out the wrong side of bed this morning' is just another way of saying that sleep affects our physical health and emotional wellbeing. Most of us know this but choose to ignore it. We don't make our sleep a priority.

Things are slowly changing, however, as research is confirming how fundamental sleep is to our overall wellbeing. Too little and poor-quality sleep are linked to various health conditions such as heart disease, high blood pressure, hormonal irregularities and suppression of the immune system function. Similarly, we know that sleep is tremendously important for our cognitive performance; for example, our alertness, attention and memory. Furthermore, sleep affects our emotional and psychological wellbeing. Sleep helps us better deal with stress, while insufficient sleep and chronic insomnia can contribute to the development of depression.

Yet these three areas are equally important in ensuring that we feel, behave and perform to the best of our abilities. In fact, physical health, cognition and emotional wellbeing relate to and influence one another, creating a triangle with equilateral sides. The triangle of wellbeing rests on sleep, as healthy sleep is a fundamental biological necessity for a healthy life.

Imagine that triangle underpinned by sleep. If your sleep becomes disrupted (I call it unhealthy) you're likely to suffer health problems, be they physical, cognitive or of an emotional nature. Our body and mind are intrinsically connected, and if one side of the health, cognition and wellbeing triangle is affected, the others are likely to become affected, too. So we can talk about a bi- or even multidirectional relationship that forms between sleep and physical health, cognitive performance and emotional wellbeing.

The following three chapters each address the relationship between sleep and one side of the triangle of health, cognition and wellbeing. I want to show you how unhealthy sleep (too short/too long and/or poor quality) impacts our health, performance and emotional wellbeing. Most research focuses on the adverse effects of unhealthy sleep, but what about the positive effects of healthy sleep? When we make it our priority to get the right amount of good-quality sleep on a regular basis, we can help reduce risks to our health and wellbeing.

# 5.

# SLEEP AND PHYSICAL HEALTH

Over the past few years, science has been revealing an ever-increasing number of physical health aspects that are impacted by sleep — in both good and bad ways. Too little sleep, sleep of poor quality and also *too much* sleep can have negative effects on your physical health and render you prone to cardiovascular disease (or CVD: an umbrella term for diseases affecting your heart and/or blood vessels; obesity, diabetes and hypertension are some of the risk factors). The right amount of sleep — which depends on your own personal sleep need — will support good health. In this chapter, we'll tour the sleep–health relationship: how sleep affects your cardiovascular system, metabolism and the major hormones involved in regulating your appetite and blood-sugar (blood-glucose) levels. Sleep also affects your eating behaviour and so it becomes an important factor in the development *and* prevention of two other increasingly common health problems: diabetes and obesity.

So let's start by looking at the sleep–diet connection.

# Gentle weight loss: a question of time and amount

Sleep affects your waistline, but how? Let's consider how sleep and eating interrelate.

Imagine coming home from work, having dinner and then preparing a few things for the next day. Then you watch some TV, and your plan is to go to bed after the news. But you change your mind when you see there's a good movie on afterwards. This means going to bed later than usual. But you reckon you'll be okay the next day even if you only get six hours' sleep instead of your usual seven. Halfway through the movie you feel peckish. So you dip into a packet of cookies; it's a big packet. By the time the film has finished and you're off to bed the packet's empty. The next evening a friend comes round. You have dinner together and while you're discussing the movie from the night before (which you both happened to watch), you start craving something sweet to eat. You remember the cake you bought earlier that day. Even though it's already 10.30 p.m. a slice of cake with a cup of tea sounds like a good idea. So not only do you have a late snack, you also have another late night with less sleep than usual. As a result, you feel quite tired the following day. For an energy boost you treat yourself to a couple of pastries for breakfast. You top up with extra coffee at 11 a.m. For a few hours it seems to work, but later that afternoon you decide to skip your usual gym class — you're just too tired. Cooking that evening seems too much of an effort, a tasty takeaway meal would be a lot easier ...

Does this story resonate with you? The occasional late-night snack or pick-me-up food because you're tired doesn't matter. But if it happens more often it can easily lead to weight gain.

There are several reasons you might gain weight. By staying up later you have extra time in which to eat. There's also *what* you eat. You've probably noticed that at night you're more likely to eat 'junk food' than a healthy salad. Studies have shown that short sleepers (i.e. those who sleep six hours or less) tend to consume fat-rich diets that are low in both protein and vegetables. Results for the intake of carbohydrates are not clear yet, but it has frequently been reported that short sleepers tend to eat more carbohydrates than do normal, healthy sleepers.

Weight gain could also be down to *eating behaviour*. Short sleepers are also more likely to eat at irregular times (that is, they tend to snack instead of having three meals at more defined times) and outside traditional eating hours. Furthermore, snacking often means eating high-calorie, energy-dense food (of lower nutritional quality) that's easy and quick to eat. Finally, snackers often continue eating after conventional dinner hours, when our metabolism is slowing down for the night. Thinking in evolutionary terms, we weren't meant to be active and eating after dark, as that would have increased the likelihood of something eating us instead!

Let's look at what other reasons there might be for gaining weight if we sleep too little. The main ones are the (potential) effects of two appetite-related hormones as well as mood-related factors.

## The dangers of being a couch potato

Two hormones, leptin and ghrelin, are involved in regulating our appetite and food intake — they influence *when* and *how much* we eat. Both of these hormones are produced and secreted within the body, leptin mainly in fat cells and ghrelin mainly in specialized stomach cells. Their signals affect the brain, in particular the hypothalamus, which is responsible for the regulation of your appetite.

Ghrelin sends the message to the brain that says you're hungry and need to eat. Its levels fluctuate during the day; they're at their highest just after midnight and then decrease until the morning. Leptin does the opposite; it signals that you're well fed and satiated. Levels of leptin are at their lowest in the morning, increasing during the day and peaking at night while we're asleep. It's the interaction of these two hormones that regulates your appetite and hunger in a way that's appropriate to the changing demands of your environment.

Several research groups have set out to investigate what happens to leptin and ghrelin when people are kept awake for longer periods or the entire night. While the exact findings are mixed, one main hypothesis is that when you stay up late at night, levels of ghrelin and leptin get out of balance. Some studies suggest that levels of ghrelin go up and levels of leptin go down. If this is true, then the altered relationship is likely to stimulate your appetite, so you become hungry and eat more during the night. Eating during the night will also confuse your stomach and body clock because this behaviour doesn't normally occur at this time.

We also need to think about energy expenditure. Ideally there's a balance between the energy we consume (i.e. our caloric intake via food) and the energy we burn while we're awake. Being physically active will draw down on our energy reserves, while eating will replenish them. In the example at the start of this chapter there was a lot of sitting down during the extra waking time. Indeed, this is what has been observed in studies on the relationship between sleep duration and activity levels. (Quick reminder: sleep duration and wakefulness are inversely related.) Habitual short sleepers (those who choose to sleep less than they need) often spend more time sitting down than normal sleepers. They're likely to have an adverse energy balance simply because they consume more calories than they burn during these extra hours awake. (Interestingly, long sleepers also spent more time being sedentary, and some studies suggest an association with weight gain. From preliminary data it seems Homer was right that 'even where sleep is concerned, too much is a bad thing'.)

The final mechanism by which short sleep might lead to weight gain is through the *hedonic* drive. (Hedonic relates to taking pleasure from something, and that pleasure then reinforces the activity/ behaviour.) The hedonic drive also involves the brain's reward system, which plays an essential role in eliciting a behaviour that is normally beneficial for survival, such as eating and drinking. The hedonic drive might be the most powerful of all mechanisms that we've discussed so far, although research around it still needs to flesh out data to conclusively confirm this.

Our reward system becomes more active in response to food when we're sleep deprived. It increases the 'value' of food in that moment. We 'want' the food, and once we've eaten we have a sense of 'liking' it, which can result in us eating even more.

Why does this happen?

It's because the brain believes we're in a survival-critical situation. Why else would we be awake and depleting our energy levels? So it promotes eating, to refill our reserves. Increasing the reward of eating makes food intake more 'attractive' to the body. So the motivation to eat is increased and we respond by eating. Unfortunately, at these times we seem to favour highly palatable, calorie-dense (and often unhealthy) food over good-quality food.

It's not only *when* we eat but also *what* we eat that can influence our sleep. Eating a diet low in fibre and high in fat and sugar can alter your sleep architecture (the stages of sleep) and how long it takes you to fall asleep. Sleep can be lighter and more disturbed, both classic signs of poor-quality sleep. Poor sleep quality will affect our cognitive abilities, such as decision-making and the reward system, the next day. This then increases the likelihood of us consuming more palatable but calorie-dense food. What you have here are the perfect ingredients for a self-perpetuating cycle of poor food choices and poor sleep — a vicious cycle.

## Diabetes

Excessive weight gain doesn't only lead to obesity. It may eventually lead to diabetes, and more specifically to type 2 diabetes. (There's some evidence suggesting that long sleep might also contribute to developing type 2 diabetes.) There are a number of different causes for developing type 2 diabetes and they differ somewhat in the mechanism of how it develops. I'll outline the pathway for diabetes caused by obesity and low physical activity, which are the triggers for the majority of cases in adults (and recently also in children).

People with diabetes have high blood glucose levels. Diabetes is a metabolic disorder, so when food is digested and subsequently used as energy it happens in a dysfunctional manner. Normally, food is broken down by the body into different nutritional groups like fat, protein and carbohydrates or sugars. Sugar enters the bloodstream as glucose, and the hormone insulin enables certain cell groups present in places like the liver, muscles and fat tissue to absorb and utilize the glucose as an energy resource. Insulin is produced by specific cells in the pancreas, so-called beta cells, in response to glucose in the blood. When the beta cells aren't able to produce enough insulin, or if the target cell groups such as muscle, fat and liver cells lose sensitivity for insulin and don't respond (a process called insulin resistance), then blood glucose levels stay elevated. If this continues, then over time (not necessarily a long time) the person enters the pre-diabetic state. This evolves into diabetes if lifestyle doesn't change.

---

A recent study showed that sleeping five hours a night for five nights reduced insulin sensitivity. The same study also looked at the recovery effects of sleep and found that three nights of nine hours' sleep a night restored insulin sensitivity, but not fully to normal levels. So for our wellbeing it's worth remembering that a weekend only gives us a maximum of two nights to recover from any potential weekday sleep loss.

---

The mechanisms by which short sleep is linked to diabetes are likely to involve many factors and include hormonal pathways and the immune system. We've already seen different examples of how sleep impacts our hormone levels; for example, with sex hormones and with appetite hormones.

Cortisol is an example of a hormonal pathway. Cortisol is a stress hormone that stimulates the liver to release stored glucose (or even produce some anew). Its main function is to get us ready and active. Levels are low during the first part of the night and begin to rise later in the second half of the sleep period, before waking up. During the day, levels of cortisol fluctuate but remain higher than at night. But by staying up longer and past your regular bedtime, cortisol levels remain higher than what is normal for this time at night. Consequently, glucose levels will be high while at the same time the sensitivity for insulin in muscular and adipose tissue might decrease.

Insulin resistance can also be caused by cells of the immune system. Short sleep elevates the levels of cytokines (or signalling molecules) that the immune system usually uses to trigger an immune reaction. Cytokines affect the sensitivity of fat, muscle and liver cells to bind insulin and, as discussed before, impair glucose uptake from the blood.

Another route linking sleep to diabetes involves the pancreatic beta cells discussed earlier. Their activity becomes reduced when we're sleep deprived and less insulin is produced. Less insulin means the signal going out to the muscle, fat and liver cells is weaker, further reducing glucose uptake by these cells.

Finally, we have the interaction of the sympathetic and parasympathetic nervous systems, also referred to as the sympatho-vagal balance.

---

The autonomic nervous system is an unconscious control system regulating our internal state (i.e. our organs and their interactions). It is divided into the sympathetic or 'fight or flight' system, and the parasympathetic 'rest and digest' system. The parasympathetic nerve fibres are bundled together in the vagus nerve, which innervates most of our bodily tissues and organs.

---

When we're asleep the activity of the sympathetic nervous system is low. The parasympathetic nervous system, on the other hand, is busy coordinating the body's repair and maintenance work, and as part of this it stimulates the secretion of insulin and promotes glucose uptake. When we're sleep deprived, however, the activity of the sympathetic system increases, getting us ready for action. Our organs become active and the release of insulin stops. That's not all, because an active sympathetic system also contributes to insulin resistance in the target tissues. Altogether, the reduction of insulin release along with the diminished sensitivity of its target tissues results in elevated blood glucose levels. And in the long-term, this leads to type 2 diabetes.

— — — — — — -

So far we've discussed the link between sleep and weight gain and obesity, as well as the link between sleep and type 2 diabetes. Diabetes and obesity are also linked and both these conditions can also *cause* sleep problems. In many cases it's not easy to work out whether insufficient sleep contributed to diabetes/obesity or if diabetes/obesity caused the poor sleep. But whichever the case, each problem or condition needs to be treated to improve overall health.

## HELPFUL HINT

Adopt a healthy lifestyle. A balanced diet, regular exercise and healthy sleep habits are vital ingredients for a healthy life. If you are concerned about your health condition, see your GP for more medical advice.

Treating type 2 diabetes and obesity is especially important since both are also risk factors for developing cardiovascular disease. And I'm sure it will come as no surprise to learn that too little, too much and poor-quality sleep are also linked to cardiovascular problems.

## Healthy sleep keeps your blood pressure in check

We've looked at the sympatho-vagal balance (or rather imbalance) and its involvement in linking short sleep and type 2 diabetes. This imbalance (i.e. the increase in the sympathetic nervous system) also plays a role in the association between short or poor sleep and the development of hypertension and heart problems. Importantly, there is also a close link between diabetes and cardiovascular disease.

The strength of this association depends to a degree on gender and, under certain circumstances, on age, too. Women who sleep too little are at higher risk than men of developing hypertension. Both genders will experience an increase in blood pressure but the mechanism to protect against acute high blood pressure reacts much faster in men than it does in women. Age seems to have an effect on extreme short sleepers (i.e. those sleeping five hours or less). Middle-aged people who fall into this sleep category are at a higher risk than all other groups. The lowest risk for developing hypertension is experienced by those sleeping seven hours a night. (It has also been suggested that long sleep may impact cardiovascular health but, as we discussed before, the mechanism isn't clear at this point.)

Like most processes in our body, blood pressure follows a circadian rhythm. Normally, blood pressure is lower at night when you're asleep compared to when you're awake during the day, although a small dip occurs in the early afternoon. There are also two peaks in its rhythm: one in the morning following awakening from sleep and one in the early evening around 7 p.m. It's the balanced and coordinated interaction of the sympathetic and the parasympathetic nervous system that's key for the regulation of the rhythm of blood pressure.

However, if we stay awake after our regular bedtime, certain parameters change. For example, we might not be in the position our body expects us to be, or we might be eating instead of fasting. While these changes themselves might affect blood pressure, insufficient sleep will lead to an activation of the sympathetic system and a deactivation of the vagal tone. Activating the sympathetic system will cause a constriction of the blood vessels (i.e. arteries and veins) and your blood pressure will go up.

I sometimes get asked about the role of magnesium and sleep. Magnesium affects the behaviour of your arteries by acting on the sympathetic system. Under normal conditions magnesium helps to dilate your arteries, making them wider and so lowering blood pressure. Not sleeping, however, decreases the concentration of magnesium in your body. This further activates the sympathetic nervous system and adds to constriction, particularly of the arteries, causing vascular tension.

Long-term vascular tension can cause chronic high blood pressure, or hypertension, which can damage your arteries by breaking their inner lining. Over time this will lead to a stiffening and thickening of the arteries. Fat from your diet then gets caught on these damaged cells and starts to clog up your arteries. This process is called atherosclerosis. Eventually these changes block the way for oxygen and nutrients going to organs such as your heart, and this can lead to serious health conditions. Further, the damaging of the vessel's inner lining, called the endothelium, is an inflammatory process that will lead to an increase in the level of cytokines, the small signalling molecules released by cells that affect communication between cells. Cytokines not only affect insulin sensitivity, but they can also affect the heart's ability to pump blood around the body. Ultimately, the heart will need to work much harder, putting it under a lot of extra strain. Which brings us to the association between sleep and the heart.

## Keep your heart healthy by sleeping well!

The heart is at the centre of your physical health. It's what keeps you alive by pumping the blood, containing oxygen and nutrients, through your body. The heart and the vascular system are closely linked; a disease affecting one will eventually affect the other. Hence conditions involving the heart and/or blood vessels are called cardiovascular diseases — these include coronary heart disease and stroke. So what's the association between sleep and the heart?

Obesity, type 2 diabetes and hypertension are all risk factors for developing cardiovascular disease. Earlier in this chapter I talked about how short and/or poor sleep increases the risk of developing each of these conditions. It's this chain of interactions or associations that links your sleep to your heart, as any of the mechanisms involved in the development of these risk factors also contributes to the risk of developing heart disease.

One aspect I haven't yet mentioned is heart rate. The rhythm of your heart rate and its variability alter across the 24-hour day.

Normally, both heart rate and variability are lower during the night while we sleep than during the day. However, the change (increase) in heart rate and variability that occurs in the early morning hours is sudden. This is mainly due to an increase in sympathetic activity — which is part of our wake-up process at the end of a normal night and so heart rate rises around the time you normally wake up. Light exposure at night has been shown to increase heart rate. The most likely reason for not going to bed at the right time (apart from suffering a sleep disorder) is that we're doing something else, for which we require light. It's this light that will then raise our heart rate for the rest of the night, even when we sleep.

When you sleep less than needed, your heart rate increases above normal levels during the following day, too. A higher heart rate increases the risk of cardiovascular disease by interacting with the other cardiovascular risk factors we have already discussed. For example, the risk of suffering a stroke or heart attack peaks between 6 a.m. and midday. This is partly due to the normal elevation in heart rate and variability that I described earlier. Another important contributing factor is blood clots, which form more easily during the night. Someone suffering from obesity and type 2 diabetes, whose arteries have become stiff and started to block up, will be far more vulnerable than a healthy person to developing blood clots.

And finally, there is the effect of moving clocks forward by an hour for daylight saving. This means losing an hour's sleep on that particular night and potentially experiencing some sleep problems on the following nights. But it also increases the risk of a heart attack by 5 per cent on the Monday and continues to stay elevated for another two days. Moving clocks back in autumn, when we gain an hour, has the opposite effect and protects us against heart attacks.

# A natural boost to the immune system

I now want to discuss the association between sleep and the immune system in more detail. Since the immune system is important in the development of cancer, I'll also highlight the link between sleep and cancer.

Lack of sleep has been shown to affect the immune response to vaccination. Not enough sleep (i.e. six hours or less, unless this really is your personal need) the nights before and/or after the vaccination can reduce the number of immune cells called antibodies needed to build immunity to the virus or bacterium at hand. Short sleep is also linked to a higher risk of catching infectious diseases such as the common cold. As with vaccination effectiveness, regularly sleeping for six hours increases your risk fourfold. Sleeping for five hours or less increases the risk by 4.5 times compared to sleeping for seven hours. (We don't yet know what the risk is for someone who's naturally a short sleeper.)

What might the underlying mechanics be? As with almost everything, the production of immune cells follows a circadian rhythm. There are many subtypes of immune cells, each having their peaks and nadirs at different times across the 24-hour day. Sleep co-regulates the number of circulating immune cells — some will go up and others will go down. For example, pro-inflammatory cytokines are released during the early part of the night to activate a slow and sophisticated immune response. On the other hand, anti-inflammatory cytokines and hormones start to be released in the late part of the night to shut down the pro-inflammatory response, and continue to be active during the day (they're responsible for an acute, fast defence against any pathogen). Not sleeping, or shortening your sleep, alters the levels of these immune cells. It shifts their peaks and nadirs, changing the internal environment of your body and making it harder for the immune system to deal with infectious agents. These effects aren't limited to nights when you're not sleeping sufficiently; they also occur during the daytime. (In a way, this is similar to what I told you about heart rate and blood pressure.) By making sleep a priority and changing or tweaking your sleep behaviour, you can therefore protect yourself better from catching diseases and give your body time to heal.

## Is there a link between sleep and cancer?

Evidence is emerging showing an association between insufficient/poor sleep and cancer, especially colorectal, prostate and breast cancers. The people most at risk are shift workers, due to their irregular sleep–wake schedules. Some studies also suggest a higher risk for those suffering from sleep apnoea (discussed in Part 3). However, more studies are needed to better understand the associations. Does sleep cause cancer and if so, how? Or does cancer cause sleep problems and if so, how? It's likely that one can lead to the other directly or indirectly, involving circadian misalignment. Disentangling the effects of sleep from the effects of the circadian system (your body clock) won't be easy, though.

# Sleep: time for your brain to get washed

Dr Maiken Nedergaard has the following delightful metaphor for how sleep allows your brain to 'clean' itself. Imagine you have a house party. And when everyone's gone home there's all that clearing up to do. Everything gets tidied up and put back in its place. But you can't do that while the party's still in full swing and you're busy being a great and entertaining host.

Something similar happens when we sleep. During the day, while we're awake and using our brain, waste material and toxic by-products of our brain's activity start to accumulate. When we're asleep the space between brain cells expands. This allows more cerebrospinal fluid to now flush through this space, washing away any toxic waste products and essentially giving the brain a proper clean-out. Quite a neat housekeeping process!

But there is something else I want to very briefly highlight here – the relationship between sleep and neurodegenerative diseases and psychiatric disorders. One of the brain's waste products is a protein called amyloid-beta. What's interesting about amyloid-beta is that it plays an important role in the development of neurodegenerative diseases such as Alzheimer's disease. In addition, many Alzheimer's patients suffer from disturbed sleep. And that brings up the question of cause and effect. Sleep might be a symptom of the disease but if it turns out that a disrupted night-time cleaning process is involved in disease progression, then sleep might be a cause of it, too.

The 'cause and effect' question' can be asked about the link between sleep and a lot of neurodegenerative diseases, as well as psychological disorders. We're only slowly beginning to understand what might be going on. One theory — which I find very exciting — proposes that sleep and normal brain function are linked via overlapping brain areas and neurotransmitters systems. (In Chapter 1, I discussed how sleep is generated in the brain using different networks and neurotransmitters.) Any alterations in these brain regions or neurotransmitter systems would then be likely to impact sleep *and* cause neurodegenerative and psychiatric disorders.

If this theory holds true, and there is research data suggesting it does, then it would offer new diagnostics and treatment options — namely, to improve sleep.

# Beauty sleep

Missing out on sleep can leave you with red, puffy eyes with dark circles under them, and pale skin. Not getting enough sleep also impacts collagen production, making your face look a little more wrinkly in the morning. An interesting study looked at the level of attractiveness of sleep-deprived people. Participants in one group had their photographs taken before and at the end of a sleep deprivation period (and were then allowed to sleep, of course). A second group, who had slept normally, were then asked to rate the photographs. Not surprisingly, the photos taken before the sleep deprivation were rated as featuring people who looked healthier and more attractive.

If you want to look attractive, make sure you get your sleep.

## To sum up

Let's recap how sleep impacts different aspects of your physical health. Short sleep can lead to weight gain; it affects your eating habits and diet. Mechanisms include a hormonal imbalance of leptin and ghrelin and the hedonic pathway, where our body rewards us for eating in order to ensure survival. We looked at how sleep is linked to insulin resistance and type 2 diabetes, conditions that are also affected by obesity. And we looked at how hypertension and the build-up of fat in the vessels can affect the heart. We reviewed the effects of sleep on the heart and the increased risk of developing cardiovascular disease when we don't get the right amount of sleep. Sleep co-regulates the immune system and influences the effectiveness of vaccinations, for example. The relationship between sleep and cancer is only just emerging but it's likely that there's a link between the two.

Sleep isn't just good for your body; it's also good for your brain and your looks. Sleep allows the brain to be cleansed and helps you to look healthy and attractive. Cause and effect between sleep and neurodegenerative and psychiatric diseases is not fully understood yet, but there's evidence that the relationship runs in both directions.

What I hope is clear after reading this chapter is that chronic sleep loss affects the body via different mechanisms or pathways, and that some of these pathways cross over and exert synergistic but damaging actions on other systems and processes in our body. Over time, this can lead to a deterioration of your physical health. And in this way, long-term sleep loss is just another form of stress you put your body under.

Good sleep, however, can help protect your health and lower your risk of diseases.

# 6.

# SLEEP WELL TO PERFORM WELL

Cognition is a rather broad term referring to a range of mental processes, and I use the terms cognition and cognitive performance interchangeably throughout this book. Cognition has to do with acquiring knowledge and understanding it — you think and perceive, make decisions and get things done. Insufficient sleep can affect how you process information, and I'm sure you know this cause-and-effect relationship from your own experience. Poor cognitive functioning can also be a symptom of neurodegenerative diseases and psychological disorders and it has been suggested that sleep might also be linked disease development and progression.

## A blow to your cognition

Concentration, decision-making, memory — these are just some of the cognitive functions we use to perform well in our day-to-day life and, from an evolutionary perspective, to survive. Many people immediately think about productivity at work when they hear the term cognitive performance, but it's not just about performance at work. It's about being able to process what's going on around us and to respond appropriately. In the face of inadequate sleep, most of us struggle to fully function the next day. Everything is done a little bit slower, and staying alert and focused requires more effort than usual.

Attention and alertness are the more 'basic' cognitive functions underlying more complex, 'executive' mental processes such as thinking, situational awareness, memory and planning. It's these two basic functions that are also the most vulnerable to sleep loss. Lack of alertness and attention slows down your reactions and responses, and you are more likely to make errors and be less accurate. Since these two are essential to all other cognitive abilities, it's clear why we see such a wide range of adverse effects on our cognitive performance when we experience prolonged sleep loss. We find it harder to learn and remember things or to think outside the box; we're less communicative (mood might play a role here, too); our awareness of what the situation demands from us is affected and often we choose ineffective solutions. Tiredness will also affect motivation, and the desire to perform well then starts to diminish.

Cognitive functions start within the brain, so it's worth asking what might be going on in the brain when we stay awake rather than go to sleep. The first brain region to be affected by sleep loss is the prefrontal cortex (PFC), an area we critically rely on for cognitive processing (Figure 6 shows you the location of the PFC in the brain). It's the reduction in metabolic activity in the PFC, which occurs with sleep loss, that's associated with reduced levels of attention and alertness. The brain then tries to compensate by recruiting other brain areas to do some of the jobs. Thus not all cognitive processes are affected at the same time and to the same degree, and you might notice an inconsistency in your performance when you're tired. Eventually, though, more and more brain areas involved in cognitive processing become affected by sleep loss. And our performance as well as cognitive flexibility and speed diminish. We're no longer able to perform consistently, appropriately and satisfactorily. Personally, I find it fascinating how actual (reversible) physiological and metabolic changes in the brain link to an observable and measurable decline in performance.

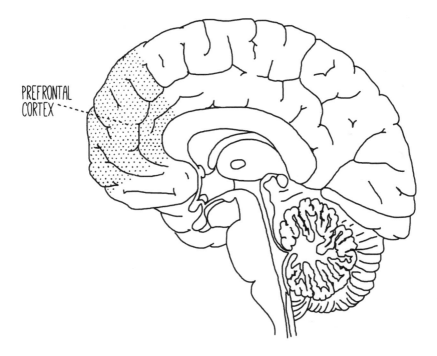

Figure 6: The brain and prefrontal cortex (PFC)

# Effects of too little sleep on the workplace

At work, a reduced cognitive performance can have serious consequences for health and safety, particularly for shift workers in safety-critical industries such as aviation, or for emergency personnel. In fact, this is the case in any situation where decision-making is critical. Fatigue is a term often used when talking about (more extreme) tiredness in the workplace. It refers to this state of reduced mental and/or physical performance due to insufficient or poor-quality sleep, being awake for too long or being awake at the 'wrong' time (wrong in the sense of your internal clock), impacting your alertness and ability to function. It's a physiological state; it can't be overcome by sheer will power. The nuclear near-melt-down of Three Mile Island in 1979, the *Challenger* Space Shuttle accident of 1986, the Chernobyl disaster in 1986, 1989's Exxon Valdez oil spill and other aviation accidents are all examples where human performance was impaired due to fatigue. In each case, workers made the wrong decision in the face of a serious problem because they struggled to assess the situation correctly. In other words, they showed less cognitive flexibility. In that way, insufficient, poor sleep became a contributing factor in causing these disasters.

But it's not just shift workers who are affected. Anyone's productivity and performance can be compromised through inadequate (i.e. insufficient and/or poor) sleep. Of those cognitive functions I mentioned earlier (and there are many more), which do you rely on in your workplace? Most if not all of them. Suppose you received an urgent request to review some data and had to make a decision on how to proceed. How much harder would it be to fully comprehend the situation and make that decision if you'd had only five hours' sleep for the previous three nights compared to being fully rested? You might need a coffee to wake you up. You might find it difficult to make sense of the information and figure out the best way forward. You might miss a crucial piece of information. Misinterpreting the data, you might make a wrong decision. I think most of us have experienced similar situations when our cognitive performance was sub-optimal due to inadequate sleep.

Sleep-deprived employees can affect a company's financial success. Productivity loss resulting from presenteeism (at work but less productive) and absenteeism (not at work) due to sleeping, on average, less than six hours is 2.4 per cent higher than when workers sleep seven to nine hours (the recommended amount of sleep). According to a recent study, that's about six working days lost per year through insufficient sleep compared to the productivity of workers who get a 'normal' amount of sleep. The same study suggests that sleep deprivation is costing the British economy £40 billion (1.86 per cent of its GDP) per year and in Germany it is £50 billion (or 1.56 per cent of its GDP). Taking into consideration the costs stemming from sleep-related health issues, it's easy to see that the implications for the economy go beyond a 'just sleep-deprived' individual. They affect the wider society and warrant asking questions about our attitude to work and its sanctity.

## Sleep and cognitive performance in your personal life

What about your personal life? To have a successful private life and to fully engage with your family and friends, the same cognitive abilities are needed. There are often problems to solve, sometimes several at the same time, requiring you to split your attention. An example might be when your children accuse each other of starting an argument — you need to be able to pay attention to what each is saying to make a 'wise' judgement. Or perhaps a friend wants to discuss with you how best to negotiate a promotion at work. Your willingness and ability to engage in a meaningful way will, among other things, depend on your cognitive processing capabilities. This is fine when you're well rested, but if you've had a few nights of poor sleep, your motivation and ability to concentrate, listen and give sound advice won't be at a level that's helpful to your friend. Which may put a strain on your friendship if your friend interprets your lack of motivation as a lack of interest in their career. Feeling hurt, they may decide not to turn to you for advice again. Equally, you might withdraw from the friendship as sleep loss is also known to affect mood (I'll come to this in the next chapter).

Do either of the two scenarios resonate with you? Can you see how your personal and social life can easily be compromised by a lack of sleep? A lot of literature looks at productivity in the workplace, but I think it's equally important to be aware of the negative effects sleep loss has on your personal life. Because that's where you really live your life.

## The internal clock and cognition

Cognitive performance isn't only influenced by the number of hours we've been awake (and, conversely, asleep). Our internal clock plays a role, too. A separate one, I should add. In Chapter 1, I showed you the circadian rhythm of alertness (see Figure 4 on p. 34) with a morning and evening peak and a small dip in the early afternoon.

Being awake at a time when your inner clock says you 'should' be asleep, as shift workers are frequently required to do, will affect your ability to concentrate. Changes to your sleep pattern — be that short, longer or disturbed sleep — will also have an effect on your internal body clock.

## We are poor judges of our own sleepiness

While reading about cognitive impairment due to lack of sleep, has a thought along the lines of 'Sleep deprivation doesn't affect me at all' crossed your mind? I ask because many people say this to me. And yes, there's variability in how well people can cope with a lack of sleep (i.e. how soon and to what degree their cognitive performance will be affected). A small number of people are more resilient to the cognitive effects of sleep loss (genetics probably play an important role here), and you might be one of them — 'the exception that proves the rule' as the saying goes. For the majority of us, though, performance and productivity suffer if we get too little sleep. The 'problem' we have as humans is that we struggle to accurately judge our own level of sleepiness. What complicates matters is that while we can easily picture and describe a drunk person, we find it harder to do so for a sleep-deprived person.

There are two interesting research studies I would like to share with you in this context. The first investigated the effects of chronic sleep loss and how it impacts your performance. Here, they also looked at how you perceive your performance when sleep deprived. (I briefly touched on this topic in Chapter 1 when answering the question 'How much sleep do I need?' on p. 26.) Participants were divided into three groups who were allowed to sleep for, respectively, a maximum of four hours, six hours or eight hours a night for fourteen nights. A fourth group didn't sleep at all for two nights. At specific times throughout the study, participants' performance was measured objectively and they were asked to rate their own level of sleepiness at the same time. The results from the performance assessment showed that scores declined across the study period: the shorter the sleep time, the worse the scores. Those sleeping six hours or less for a prolonged time (in this case, fourteen nights) showed comparable performance degradation with those not sleeping at all for two nights.

What about the subjective sleepiness ratings? For the first four days, participants said that their sleepiness was increasing slightly, which matched their decline in performance. But then their ratings plateaued and participants said they did not get any sleepier — despite missing out on even more sleep. What was going on? Did they adapt to the lack of sleep? No, they didn't. As I told you, when measured objectively performance continued to decline across the fourteen days. What had changed was their sense of their own sleepiness and their ability to judge it accurately.

The three key messages from this study are:

+ Over time, even a small to moderate decrease in sleep duration can cause the same decline in performance as a whole night with no sleep.

+ People don't adapt to insufficient sleep. Many of us for one reason or another only sleep for six hours, which may be enough for some but the majority of us need at least seven hours.

+ We're poor judges of our own sleepiness. We get used to feeling tired, thinking we've adapted to less sleep. It's almost as if we lose the sense for feeling how sleepy we really are. We think we're as productive as ever, that we're performing at our best, when in reality our cognitive performance is reduced.

The other study I want to highlight was undertaken by researchers Dawson and Reid in 1997. Sleep deprivation was shown to affect performance in a similar way to alcohol. Study participants were given alcohol at set intervals until their blood alcohol concentration (BAC) had reached 0.10 per cent. A week later, the same participants were kept awake for 28 hours. During both trials, participants had to complete a performance test every half-hour. Not surprisingly, performance declined on both occasions. What's really interesting, though, is that after being awake for seventeen hours the level of cognitive impairment was *equivalent* to that when blood alcohol concentration had reached 0.05 per cent (the legal drink driving limit in Australia and most European countries) and when participants were starting to get drunk. Being awake for seventeen hours is considered a moderate level of sleep deprivation because it still leaves a maximum of seven hours for sleep (or time in bed, I should say). How much sleep are you getting on a regular basis?

- - - - - - - - - - - - - - - - - - - - - - - - -

Blood alcohol levels can vary widely between people, depending on factors such as gender and body weight. While person A might reach a BAC of 0.1 per cent after drinking four standard beers (that's just over 1 litre, or almost 2½ pints), person B might be able to drink seven beers (equivalent to around 2 litres, or just over 4 pints) before reaching the same BAC.

- - - - - - - - - - - - - - - - - - - - - - - - -

Think of a time when you were tipsy. Were you able to hold a conversation and be aware of what was going on around you? Now compare that to engaging in a conversation after a poor night's sleep. Different? Similar?

I think the results from this second study show the effects of sleep deprivation on our performance and that they're real. Sacrificing your sleep won't make you more successful — either professionally or personally. But there's one thing you can do to enhance your success. Sleep. It's *the* most natural performance booster.

- - - - - - - - - - - - - - - - - - - - - - - - - -

A well-known example of how cognition might impact sleep is repetitive negative thinking and worrying. A lot of people say that worrying about work and personal life issues is what keeps them awake at night. Or they lie there ruminating about the past. You might even have experienced this yourself. I'll go into more detail about this in Chapter 7, where we'll discuss sleep and stress.

- - - - - - - - - - - - - - - - - - - - - - - - - -

## To sum up

In this chapter, we've explored how inadequate (insufficient/poor) sleep can negatively affect your cognitive performance and I've explained what we think is happening in the brain of a sleep-deprived person. Lack of sleep is associated with lower productivity in the workplace and can affect your problem-solving skills in your personal life. Worrying and repetitive thinking, on the other hand, have the ability to disturb your sleep (which in turn can impair your cognitive performance).

# 7.

# EMOTIONAL WELLBEING AND SLEEP

Emotional wellbeing is the balance of both positive and negative moods and emotion. (I will use mood and emotion interchangeably, putting aside for now the subtle difference between them.) It's when you're fully able to deal with both the ups and downs of your life and function in society. Emotional wellbeing and sleep are closely connected. Insufficient, but more so poor quality, sleep at night impacts your emotional functioning the following day, while being anxious during the day alerts the mind, which isn't ideal when you want to sleep.

In this chapter I'll discuss both sides of the 'sleep and emotional wellbeing' relationship and how this can sometimes turn into a vicious cycle of poor sleep and negative emotions.

# The doom and gloom that follows a short night

'Why's everyone so irritating today? What's wrong with them? Hmm, hang on, maybe it's me who's the grumpy one. I did go to bed quite late last night because of the theatre show and the drinks afterwards.'

Sound familiar? Yes, it's quite likely that you're actually the grumpy one. Inadequate sleep not only decreases positive mood and emotions while increasing and intensifying negative mood and emotions; it also diminishes your ability to self-monitor your emotional state along with your ability to appropriately engage with your partner, friends or colleagues, because you struggle to accurately 'read' facial expressions and perceive their emotions correctly and respond empathetically. Instead, we're more likely to blame others for things that go wrong and become more irritable, distressed and angry. Next, we start growing more and more anxious, thinking the worst-case scenario is definitely going to happen.

But it doesn't stop there. After a poor night's sleep our impulse control is reduced, which can have serious consequences, especially in the workplace! Imagine you have a conflict at work. Let's say you disagree with your boss's opinion about a report you've written. When you're fully rested, you behave in a way that aims to resolve the conflict. You fully comprehend the situation (you are in charge of your cognitive functions) and you're aware of your emotions (after all, *you* have written this report). However, in a sleep-deprived state objectivity goes out of the window and a red mist descends. You become frustrated and more likely to make hostile comments in your communication with your boss and others. You might even send out emails you later regret. On top of that, you couldn't care less about the potential repercussions of your behaviour because you're only able to focus on the negative things in front of you —

your boss's disagreement, which to you is unacceptable in this moment. As you can see, inadequate sleep increases negative moods and impairs emotional processing. This inability to regulate your emotions and mood can impact your relationships, potentially leading to serious adverse consequences such as the end of a personal or professional relationship.

## Is a lack of sleep killing your motivation?

Our motivation to get things done and to engage with others is diminished when we don't get enough sleep over a longer period of time. How we evaluate rewards changes, too. We go for quick but small wins rather than large rewards that require more effort. So instead of going to your evening gym class, which you know will be a bit arduous but you'll feel great afterwards, you go straight home after work to slouch on the sofa and watch TV. You feel grumpy and sluggish after two nights of poor sleep and simply can't face up to the challenge. All you want is to just rest and for your emotional needs to be met immediately and as easily as possible. But how might you feel the next morning, having had no exercise or a catch-up with your gym friends the evening before? Probably annoyed and disappointed with yourself.

The danger is that we can get into a vicious cycle by avoiding challenging situations like professional meetings and social activities. In the short term it might reduce negative emotions and leave you feeling relieved. But in the longer term it can lead to isolation and feelings of loneliness and inadequacy. It may reinforce low mood and motivation and perpetuate inactivity. You might even stop engaging with friends and work colleagues. Compare that with the fun of being active, meeting friends and feeling good about yourself the morning after.

But not going to the gym is not only about feeling disappointed. Not doing regular exercise (while also enjoying energy-rich 'food for the soul') can also lead to weight gain and obesity. And how that can affect your sleep you already know from reading Chapter 5. If you haven't, then I suggest you read it next.

## Losing your neutrality

Emotional and cognitive processes interact and underpin our mental state. Both are affected by sleep loss, and any impairment of one system will impact the other. Let's take attention as an example of this interaction. When we are well rested we intentionally focus our attention on somebody or something and then direct our attention onto another stimulus, and the next and the next. At times, this shift in attention can help regulate our emotions, because we purposely divert our attention from a negative emotional stimulus towards something positive or neutral. However, when you're sleep deprived, deliberately shifting your attention becomes more and more difficult (as we've already discussed in the previous chapter on cognition and performance).

But it's not just our ability to direct our attention that's influenced by sleep loss. Several studies have suggested, and you may know this from personal experience, that we tend to focus more on negative rather than positive stimuli. It's almost as if we're looking for negative information. Some of these research studies have used emotional faces to investigate attention. Measuring participants' brain activity as they responded, they found that while attention to negative, threat-related faces (those portraying anger or fear, for example) created a normal or heightened neural response, positive or neutral faces create a much smaller neural response in the brain. In a sleep-deprived state this difficulty in understanding another's emotions is even more heightened, which often creates tension and leads to frustration. But it's not all doom and gloom after inadequate sleep. Sometimes we experience the exact opposite: we have moments of (perhaps unseemly) elation and excitement.

A possible explanation for these two somewhat opposing observations is that lack of sleep intensifies emotional processing (of negative as well as positive stimuli) and creates an effective imbalance. One research group conducted a study to further investigate the mechanisms of the emotional impairment we experience if we don't get enough sleep. They deprived participants of sleep for one night, and revealed fascinating results. In addition to intensifying the processing of emotional stimuli, sleep loss also impacted the processing of neutral stimuli. What's more, participants were easily distracted regardless of the type of stimuli (emotional or neutral) when sleep deprived. (Fully rested participants, however, were only distracted by emotional stimuli.) Simultaneous brain scans revealed a change of activity in the amygdala, our emotional centre and evolutionary threat radar. (See Figure 7 for where in the brain the amygdala is located.) This brain region normally only reacts in response to salient emotional stimuli, but when participants were bleary eyed it reacted to *all* incoming events, regardless of the emotional value.

This study tells us that without sleep the brain loses its ability to ignore irrelevant information. Suddenly everything becomes important because the threshold for emotional activation is lowered. As a result, we lose our neutrality and everything gets out of proportion. Cognitive processing might become biased, affecting our ability to judge, which in itself can lead to increased anxiety levels. The smallest thing can cause us to lose our temper. Interestingly, even the pitch, energy and sharpness of our voice changes and we sound sadder and more stressed.

As maladaptive and misplaced as such behaviour certainly is, theoretically there might be an evolutionary advantage in being worried and irritable in response to sleep loss. Being biased and anxious towards an unfamiliar stimulus puts us into a position from which we can quickly react and so protect ourselves against a potential threat.

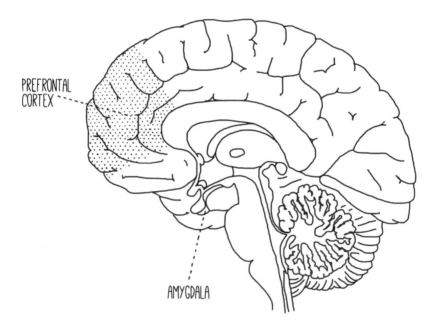

Figure 7: The amygdala and prefrontal cortex

The amygdala is part of the limbic system and is involved in the processing of emotional stimuli. True to the motto 'better safe than sorry', the amygdala views most events or stimuli in a negative light to make sure we survive. But that also can lead to elevated anxiety and stress levels.

# Feeling grumpy in the morning: a matter of connectedness

The *medial* prefrontal cortex (mPFC) is a region within your executive brain centre that's believed to be responsible for the monitoring and regulation of the amygdala. If left unchecked, the negativity bias and innate tendency of the amygdala to register an event as potentially harmful can trigger a defensive, and at times inappropriate, response.

Perceiving a threat (real or imagined) will trigger the body's stress response, also called the fight or flight response. It is a survival mechanism that enables us to quickly react and either fight or run away from danger. However, the amygdala sometimes overreacts and responds to non-threatening daily life events, such as a busy commute or giving an important presentation, putting the body into a state of hyper-arousal which will make falling or staying asleep more difficult.

The job of the mPFC is to analyze an event in more detail and to initiate an appropriate behavioural response so we don't overreact. An example might be if you hear what you think is a mouse, are about to jump, then realize the sound was simply a falling leaf and continue walking.

However, things change when we're sleep deprived. In Chapter 6, I discussed how sleep loss affects the PFC and how this impacts your ability to think clearly. What's of importance here is that the lack of (good) sleep reduces the functional connectivity between the mPFC and amygdala. It weakens the regulatory influence of the mPFC over your emotional responses. As a result, the amygdala can now 'run around like an unruly child' and shout 'danger', 'doom and gloom'. And so you become more emotionally reactive but less able to respond appropriately to the demands of your environment.

When discussing the effects of sleep loss on cognitive performance, we looked at how people can vary in their susceptibility to the effects of poor or insufficient sleep. The same applies when it comes to emotional functioning and sleep deprivation. You may have already noticed it: perhaps your partner's a bit quiet after a late night while you, on the other hand, fly off the handle at the smallest thing when you haven't had enough sleep. There's also scientific evidence suggesting that women are more susceptible than men to negative emotions following a poor night. Whether there are also differences between age groups hasn't yet been investigated but it's likely to be the case.

## REM sleep and emotions

Researcher Eti Ben Simon and colleagues found something else in their study that's of interest here, concerning REM sleep. In Chapter 1, I mentioned the special role REM sleep plays in the consolidation of emotional memories. In addition, it might also be that REM sleep modulates our (extreme) emotional experiences by altering and diminishing the intensity of their emotional tone. Ultimately it seems that REM sleep supports an adaptation of our behaviour. (It's about us being better prepared and able to respond appropriately the next time we encounter a similar situation.) Abnormalities in REM sleep, however, are associated with alterations in daytime mood. What Simon and colleagues found, as have others before them, is that a diminished connectivity between the mPFC and amygdala is associated with lower amounts of REM sleep. During REM sleep, a specific neurotransmitter called noradrenaline is inhibited to allow for proper functioning of both the mPFC and amygdala. Lack of REM therefore keeps noradrenaline concentrations high. This prevents the mPFC from doing its job of controlling the amygdala and ensuring a balance in our emotional reactivity the next day. To sum up, sleep and particularly REM sleep are important for overnight processing and next-day regulation of your emotions.

You might be wondering if it's easy to miss out on REM sleep. I think it is. The most common 'form' of sleep loss in our society is that caused by late, short nights. Although we still get the SWS-rich sleep, the amount of REM sleep we experience is reduced since we get most of our REM sleep in the latter part of our sleep. By getting up early the next day to go to work, we particularly cut short the part of our sleep that is rich in REM. See how easy it is? Drinking alcohol makes it even worse! Alcohol makes you fall asleep faster and have more deep sleep during the first sleep cycles, which comes at the cost of your REM sleep. Particularly during the second part of the night, with its REM-rich sleep cycles, alcohol's effect on the body (toilet trips, thirst, snoring) wakes you up and disturbs your sleep. Some researchers therefore think that the hangover and grumpy mood the next day are to some extent the result of too little REM sleep. If you get the chance to nap in the morning after a heavy night you'll enter REM sleep much quicker than the usual 90 minutes because your body's lacking what it didn't get during the night.

> Good sleep will support your emotional wellbeing
> and will help you to be more balanced and better
> at noticing and regulating your emotions the next
> day. Perhaps one function of sleep is to provide
> us with some free therapy hours.

# Emotions and their impact on sleep

We've looked at how sleep affects your emotions. Now let's consider the other side of the relationship: how emotions affect sleep. Negative emotions such as anxiety, unhappiness and sadness can disturb our sleep in the night/s preceding or following an emotional event. Suppose you have a big meeting to attend at work or a talk to give the next morning — how well do you sleep the night before? Or how well do you think you would sleep after having a huge argument with your best friend?

Many people report troubles falling or staying asleep and studies using polysomnography have shown that emotional stress impacts various aspects of our sleep and its architecture. Studies differ in respect to their findings; some studies have reported a reduction in sleep duration and efficiency. This is due to more awakenings, changes in REM sleep and dreaming. Other research groups didn't find any changes in REM sleep but confirmed the impact on total sleep time and noted that it took their participants longer to enter deep sleep. Interestingly, and in line with the previous point on the role of REM sleep, alterations in

REM sleep are more frequently observed than in NREM sleep. Some studies report no sleep disturbance but instead longer than usual sleep duration following stressful events. (Although this might be viewed as positive, it's still a change from normal sleep behaviour.) Positive emotions, on the other hand, seem to have a positive effect on sleep. As inconsistent or limited as all of these results might be, they confirm what many of us experience ourselves: emotional experiences during the day often impact our sleep the following night/s.

This doesn't mean that every emotionally negative situation causes sleep disturbances or that everyone will experience problems sleeping following such an event. The type and intensity of the emotionally stressful event and how well you're able to process and regulate your emotions seem to play a role here. If you haven't fully processed your emotions during the waking hours — perhaps the event happened too close to bedtime or it was highly stressful — this processing might continue during the night, interfering with your sleep. Think of an unfinished piece of work and how it stays in your mind until it's dealt with.

## HELPFUL HINT

How you respond to an emotional experience and what coping style you use to deal with it are additional factors influencing the impact emotions have on your sleep. Turning towards your negative emotions, accepting and expressing them will help to better process them. Problem-solving strategies also involve turning towards the event, but here it's about analyzing what caused the event and what its consequences are.

A third type of coping style is to avoid or disengage from emotional stress by the use of denial and suppression strategies, as if withdrawing from being awake and 'escaping' to sleep. (This type of behaviour helps explain findings where sleep duration was extended.) Which of the different coping strategies is most beneficial might depend on the type of stressor you are experiencing in that moment rather than the rigid use of a specific coping style. Adopting a flexible approach when dealing with difficult emotions might prove most advantageous.

## Stress: how cognition and emotion interact to affect sleep

Experiencing stress is unpleasant. We perceive something as stressful when we feel unable to meet the demands the environment or situation places on us. Work-related stress is probably the most common stressor we experience in our modern society. If the stress is short-term, the body and mind have time to recover and it's not harmful. In fact, short-term stress might help us get things done. If work-related stress isn't resolved and persists it turns into chronic stress. This starts to deplete our energy resources, affecting our health and wellbeing.

Regardless of whether it is short-term or chronic, stress can disturb your sleep, leaving you feeling emotionally drained and cognitively and physiologically exhausted the next day. But it's not so much the stress that causes the sleep problems; it's how you cope with feeling stressed that will have the bigger influence on your sleep. Are you able to let go of the stress and leave it at work, for example, or are you taking it home with you?

Leisure time is what helps us to wind down and detach from work-related stress. It's a time when we do things such as go to the gym, play with our children or see friends, to switch off from work. This allows our brain and body to recover and our energy sources to replenish. However, if we cut our leisure time by working late, if we don't manage to disengage mentally from the work stressors and ruminate about unfinished work stuff, if we spend our time anticipating and worrying about what we have on the next day, we stay cognitively stimulated. This in turn will keep our stress system, including the amygdala, activated and we become physiologically aroused, too. (Have you ever noticed your heart pumping faster, your chest feeling tight, your shoulders and neck tensing up, feeling hot or sweaty? These are all signs of the stress response.) Once you're in this state of hyper-arousal, sleeping becomes 'naturally' more difficult.

The stress response is trying to help us in a life-threatening situation. Would you want to fall asleep when you're in danger? And even if you do fall asleep, because the amygdala and the stress system never really shut down for the night, they're ready to hijack those brief awakenings at the end of a sleep cycle. Then you're back to ruminating and worrying — and back to not sleeping.

## Rumination and worry

Repetitive thinking (or cognitive arousal) activates the stress response (physiological arousal), which puts the body and mind into a hyper-alert state. However, it's unlikely that thoughts from cognitive stressors, such as rumination and worry, occur in isolation from emotions and emotional arousal. Rumination is closely linked to feeling low and angry, while worrying is associated with feeling anxious.

Rumination and worry are two behaviours most of us will engage in from time to time. Rumination is the repetitive thinking about past problematic events and the emotions evoked by these events. Worry, on the other hand, is more about future concerns. (By the way, we fear far more events than actually happen.) Both drive cognitive arousal and have been associated with poor sleep quality and a longer sleep latency.

Worry includes problem-solving, another cognitive process that can interfere with sleep. Why? It is a behaviour that should be short-term because either a solution is found or the problem is put aside for the time being (e.g. when going to bed). But if this is not the case, the problem-solving continues, eventually turning into worry. Many people do not perceive this as worrying, yet it is something that your mind continues to work on (cognitive arousal).

Maybe you've noticed that lying there at night ruminating about the day's events or worrying about work the next day can make you feel a little upset or anxious. It is these emotions that will further activate your amygdala, intensifying the hyper-arousal you're experiencing. The way work stress can affect us is a compelling example of how cognitive and emotional arousal interact and affect your sleep.

Taking a broader perspective and looking beyond the effects of stress, cognitive and emotional arousal could form a vicious cycle. Negative emotions trigger negative thoughts, which disturb sleep, while negative thoughts might further amplify negative emotions, making sleep harder to come by or disrupting it. It's also possible that everything starts with poor sleep — that inadequate sleep can trigger a negative mood and (repetitive) thoughts that are detrimental to sleep. When taking steps to improve your sleep, perhaps being aware of this complex relationship might be more important that understanding *how* this vicious cycle has formed. Trying to acknowledge this, rather than becoming absorbed by the unpleasant and unwanted thoughts and emotions, will help you to get back to a restful night. (See Chapter 14 for more help on how to respond to unwanted thoughts and emotions.)

## To sum up

In this chapter we looked at both sides of the relationship between sleep and emotional wellbeing. Inadequate sleep influences how we feel during the day. After one or two poor nights, we're likely to become irritable and anxious, often hitting out at the people closest to us both in our personal and professional lives. Emotions we experience during the waking day, on the other hand, can influence how well we sleep. Current research suggests that REM sleep in particular is important for emotional processing. We all use different strategies to cope with difficult emotions, and which strategies work best may depend on the situation and the stressor. When we feel stressed this often disturbs our sleep. Rumination and worry are cognitive processes closely linked to negative emotions, which reinforce one another and keep you in a hyper-aroused state when instead you would like to sleep.

You might notice that in this chapter I did not talk much about positive emotions and sleep. This is because research on sleep naturally focuses on the negative effects of sleep rather than how and why things go right. Looking more closely at how and why things go right — at how, for example, positive emotions and a healthy lifestyle support good sleep — will inform the development of future therapies and coping strategies for disturbed sleep.

# part 3

*

# WHEN SLEEP GOES WRONG

+

- - - - - - - - - - -

Dear mother of fresh thoughts and joyous health!

William Wordsworth, 1806

In the previous section we looked at the effects of inadequate sleep on health and wellbeing. We'll now take a more detailed look at sleep disorders. It doesn't matter whether it's a sleep disorder or your lifestyle that causes poor or short sleep; insufficient sleep is a health and wellbeing hazard.

I decided to go into detail in this section because I think there are many people suffering from a sleep disorder without being aware of it. They may feel tired and struggle to get through the day, their cognitive performance may be impaired and their mood low or grumpy. However, because they don't know what healthy sleep actually is, and its relevance for health and wellbeing, they don't seek help. Or if they do, their health care professional might lack awareness about sleep and not know how to screen for sleep disorders.

I hope that by reading the following chapters you'll get a good understanding of the symptoms of the different sleep disorders so that if you notice them in yourself, your partner or a friend, you'll seek advice and have an informed discussion with your GP. I suggest you also ask for a full medical check-up, as many health conditions such as thyroid disease, the side-effects of certain medications, vitamin B12 deficiency and food allergies are often associated with sleep problems.

## Categories of sleep disorders

Somnipathy is the scientific term for a medical disorder of sleep patterns. There are over 100 sleep disorders that regularly lead to complaints about too little sleep or too much sleep.

Thankfully, sleep experts have grouped them into six major categories, as outlined in the following table.

## Major categories of sleep disorders

| 1. Sleep-related breathing disorders | 2. Sleep-related movement disorders | 3. Chronic insomnia disorders |
|---|---|---|
| Difficulty breathing during sleep | Simple, unwanted, often repetitive movements during sleep | Trouble falling or staying asleep, waking up too early, or not feeling refreshed in the morning despite adequate sleep |
| **4. Hypersomnias** | **5. Parasomnias** | **6. Circadian rhythm sleep–wake disorders** |
| Excessive daytime sleepiness interfering with day-to-day life | Abnormal behaviours or movements during sleep | Sleep times are misaligned with the environment |

In this section, we'll look at some of the most prevalent sleep disorders. Some can have severe consequences for health and wellbeing. Note that this isn't a comprehensive review; I want to raise awareness of these disorders, their signs and symptoms, so that you're better equipped to notice a potential sleep disorder in yourself (or your bedfellow) and are empowered to have an informed discussion with your GP or sleep specialist.

---

Not every sleep problem is a sign of a sleep disorder. Two weeks of poor sleep in response to a stressful event isn't unusual, but if you feel unrefreshed and struggle to perform during the day, or you find you are emotionally fragile outside of a stressful period, this could suggest a sleep disorder. The resources in 'Further reading' (p. 213) provide additional sources of information on sleep disorders.

---

# 8.

# SLEEP-RELATED BREATHING AND MOVEMENT DISORDERS

## Sleep-related breathing disorders

George's wife Erica had told him many times that over the past couple of years he would stop breathing several times during the night. It was something that frightened her — after a period of absolute silence, when only his abdominal wall was moving, he would suddenly take in a huge, and very loud, gasp of air. It was this loud noise that disrupted her sleep almost every night, sometimes making her feel irritable in the morning. George didn't seem to wake up, or at least not knowingly. But when he noticed that he felt very tired during the day, and struggled more and more with cognitively challenging tasks, George finally decided to see his GP. It didn't take the GP long to diagnose a sleep-related breathing disorder. The treatment plan the GP devised together with George included changes to his lifestyle and wearing a breathing device at night to allow a proper flow of oxygen. Although it took George over a year to get used to his device, he soon started to notice how much better he felt during the day, and how not only his but also Erica's sleep quality improved.

Sleep-related breathing disorders arise when you experience difficulties breathing or even pause breathing during your sleep. There are 3 important types of these disorders that I'll discuss in more detail. I'll start with obstructive sleep apnoea (OSA), which is what George was diagnosed with. Apnoea refers to a complete cessation of airflow.

## Obstructive sleep apnoea

Obstructive sleep apnoea (OSA) is the most common sleep-related breathing disorder. New estimates expect that 34 per cent of men and 17 per cent of women aged between 30 and 70 have it. Interestingly, prevalence rates don't differ very much between countries, making OSA a global health problem. Often it is undiagnosed and therefore untreated with potentially severe effects on an individual's health.

In OSA, the muscles of your upper airway collapse, and while you try to breathe (when your abdominal wall extends) none or only a limited amount of air can reach your lungs. In some people, the limited airflow makes the throat tissue vibrate, leading to snoring. If you don't breathe properly, blood oxygen levels decrease and carbon dioxide levels increase. The brain notices this as an emergency situation and sends a signal to arouse you. While you may not necessarily wake up fully, you'll wake enough to take in a deep breath of air that appears as a loud snore or noisy gasp before you slip back into light sleep.

The problem is that these repeated micro-arousals will disrupt your sleep and stop you from getting sufficient deep sleep. It's a bit like diving underwater for a fixed period of time; without an oxygen tank you have to keep coming up to the surface to get air and so can't really explore what's far beneath you. Poor sleep quality, morning headaches and excessive daytime sleepiness are direct consequences of this unrestful and unrestorative sleep. Excessive tiredness during the day can lead to uncontrolled and unplanned naps — anytime, anywhere. Drivers are particularly at risk because they could fall asleep while behind the wheel and cause an accident. You might also feel irritable and find it hard to concentrate and perform at work. But it doesn't stop there. OSA increases your risk of cardiovascular and metabolic diseases such as diabetes and hypertension. And it might affect your libido! Most OSA sufferers are unaware of their condition and it's their partner or their compromised mental and physical health that eventually leads them to consult a sleep specialist.

Who's at risk? Well, OSA is associated with being overweight and a loss of muscle tone in the upper airways. Middle-aged men carrying some extra pounds and with a collar size of 43 centimetres (17 inches) or more, and also postmenopausal women (as discussed in Chapter 3, ovarian hormone levels decrease and the chance of weight gain increases) are therefore the ones most at risk. Older age is another risk factor, but because of the current rise in child obesity, more and more children experience OSA, too, affecting their physical and mental growth. Lifestyle factors also contribute to OSA. Alcohol and sedatives, for example, relax the muscles of the upper airways. Physical features such as large tonsils or a small jaw bone or chin, or your genetics can also increase your risk of OSA.

The good news is that OSA is treatable and there are many different options. For example, there are oral appliances such as mandibular advancement devices, and continuous positive airway pressure (CPAP) devices that can help you breathe better.

---

A lot of people struggle with their CPAP because they find it hard to wear the mask all night. Instead of ditching your treatment strategy, talk to your GP about the difficulties you're experiencing so that together you can find a workable solution. Sometimes it might just be a matter of getting used to the treatment. Admittedly that may take a long time, but remember what's at stake — your health and performance as well as your partner's sleep and wellbeing.

---

Other therapy devices help you to reposition yourself during your sleep without waking you up. Surgery is another option, but often not very effective. Talk to your GP or sleep specialist about what strategy makes sense to help you. And finally, but perhaps most importantly, adopt a healthy lifestyle.

## Central sleep apnoea

Central sleep apnoea (CSA) is similar to OSA but less common. With CSA you also repeatedly stop breathing, but this is because your body doesn't make the effort to breathe (unlike with OSA, where you have an obstructed upper airway).

There are many different reasons this happens. There could be a problem in generating the drive to breathe, almost as if your brain 'forgets' to send the signal to breathe. Or it might be that your breathing muscles are too weak. Crucially, and similar to OSA, when you stop breathing, blood oxygen levels start to fall and levels of carbon dioxide accumulate. The high levels of carbon dioxide trigger you to breathe again, which you do with ease because nothing's blocking your airways. But the problem with these breathing interruptions is that they're associated with a brief arousal where you may not wake up fully, but your sleep is nevertheless interrupted and won't be as restorative as it should and could be. So the next day you feel tired, struggle to perform and might be grumpy. If CSA persists, it can also affect your cardiovascular health. But, here again, several treatment options are available and are very often the same as those used to treat OSA.

Finally, CSA symptoms might also occur at altitudes above 2000 metres (6500 feet) where less oxygen is available. As soon as you've acclimatized, your breathing will improve and the CSA will disappear.

## Snoring

Snoring is the loud, coarse sound that results from air turbulence inside the airway when you breathe in. I'm sure you know it. It happens when the muscles in the back of your mouth, throat and tongue relax and constrict or obstruct the airway. This causes the soft tissue in the nose, mouth or throat to vibrate, leading to that well-known snoring sound.

Generally speaking, snoring is more common in men (40 per cent) than in women (24 per cent) and is more likely to occur in older than in younger people. Body weight is also a risk factor for snoring; there's a correlation between a higher BMI and snoring. Interestingly, for most habitual snorers it's their sleeping position that triggers the snoring. You may have noticed that sleeping on the back causes you (or your partner) to snore. You might also have noticed that alcohol and other substances or medications that make your throat muscles relax make snoring more likely.

What are the consequences of snoring? Most of all, it's a nuisance to all who have to hear it. Light snoring is the most common 'type' of snoring, and can leave you with a dry mouth or throat but not much more. Heavy snoring, however, can be a symptom of OSA and if left untreated can lead to many serious health conditions. If you often find yourself extremely tired during the day despite adequate sleep, and if you or your partner notice you gasping for air at night, that could be a sign that you're suffering from sleep apnoea. Speak to your GP or sleep specialist about it if you're concerned, and find the best treatment options.

# Sleep-related movement disorders

This is a group of sleep disorders that cause you to move before or even during sleep. Falling or staying asleep can be a real struggle at times, and peaceful sleep recedes into the distance. Daytime performance and emotional wellbeing will also be affected. The movements themselves are typically simple and stereotyped, which is also what differentiates these disorders from the movements seen in other sleep disorders and normal sleep.

## Restless legs syndrome

Restless legs syndrome (RLS) is a neurological or sensorimotor disorder where you have a strong urge to move mainly your legs. You can also experience very uncomfortable, unpleasant sensations in your legs. Perhaps some of these words will resonate with you to describe the sensations you experience in the evening and during the night: painful, creepy crawly, tugging or itching. Many people say that they feel these unpleasant sensations deep within their thigh or calf muscles, or even the whole leg.

The symptoms usually start in the evening as you begin to relax, and just after midnight is when they're at their worst. Then it really feels like worms are creeping in your legs, keeping you awake for a few hours or sometimes all night. What can help is to move or walk. But the symptoms can return as soon as you rest again. And so your sleep becomes more fragmented and disturbed, and you feel fatigued during the day.

In addition to these symptoms, you might also experience periodic limb or leg movements during your sleep, specifically during NREM sleep, but also when you lie down to rest in the evening. Your leg muscles tighten or flex but, crucially, these movements are beyond your control, which makes them even more annoying.

People of any age can develop RLS, yet it's people over the age of 45, and in particular women, who are more at risk than others. The gender bias is in part due to the fact that up to 30 per cent of pregnant women suffer from RLS during their last trimester of pregnancy. Other causes for RLS include low iron levels, genetics and problems with the dopamine-signalling pathway in the brain.

Factors contributing to RLS are medical conditions such as diabetes or Parkinson's disease, medication and, of course, lifestyle. There's currently no cure for RLS, only ways to manage it better. Apart from pharmacological treatment, lifestyle changes and mindfulness-based therapies can help to increase quality of life.

## Periodic limb movements disorder

Periodic limb movements disorder (PLMD) is a condition where involuntary, repetitive and stereotyped limb movements disturb your sleep and cause you to feel unrefreshed and excessively tired the next day. PLMs can happen while you're awake resting or during your sleep. They're very common and everyone can have them from time to time during their sleep. Typically, you're not aware of them because the movements are small and don't cause you to wake up. As such, they're benign and not considered a disorder unless they interrupt your sleep and severely affect your everyday life.

PLMD can affect anyone and any age group; however, the older you are the higher the risk. The cause for PLMD isn't known and unfortunately there's no cure for it. But because of its close link to RLS, some of the same drugs can be used to manage the symptoms to give you some relief.

– – – – – –

Other sleep-related movements disorders include bruxism, where you clench or grind your teeth, and 'sleep starts' or hypnic jerks, which occur as you're falling asleep (see p. 19). To learn more, please see the Further reading list on p. 213.

# 9.

# CHRONIC INSOMNIA DISORDER

Insomnia is Latin for 'want of sleep' or 'sleeplessness'. Both translations hit the proverbial nail on the head, highlighting the core problem of the disorder: the inability to sleep while at the same time wanting nothing but sleep.

As you can imagine, or perhaps know from first-hand experience, there are different 'ways' you might experience sleep problems. Insomnia *disorder* is therefore used as an umbrella term to describe quite a complex condition. There are different types which may or may not change within a person, different classifications based on how long you've had the symptoms, differences in severity which can also change within a person, and finally insomnia can be its own disorder or a symptom of another sleep or medical condition. To give you an example of the heterogeneity of insomnia, when I ask clients to describe their symptoms they complain about having troubles falling or staying asleep, or waking up too early, or (but this seems much rarer) they just don't feel refreshed in the morning but don't complain about a problem with sleeping as such. Some will list one or two symptoms which they've had for years, while others say their insomnia evolved and their symptom/s changed over the past few months. Others may experience different combinations of symptoms. These symptoms might happen every night or come in cyclic bouts. Factor in varying durations and causes and the assessment can get very complex.

There are three types of insomnia. If you have repeated problems falling asleep you experience *sleep onset insomnia*. If you struggle to stay asleep and keep waking up during the night it is called *sleep maintenance insomnia*. And if you wake up too early in the morning it's sometimes called terminal insomnia, a term I don't use as it suggests there's no hope of ever sleeping normally again, which isn't true; so instead let's refer to it as *waking up too early*.

Irrespective of when during the night you cannot sleep, it usually doesn't take long before your mind starts racing. You worry about not sleeping and how this will affect your performance the next day. 'Will I be able to give my presentation and talk coherently?' you might think. Or you lie there ruminating, analyzing the past day and what you could have said instead of a begrudging 'No problem' when a grumpy barista spilled coffee over your new coat. Or you might think, 'I don't worry, I just go through my to-do list and other life admin', which in a way is just the same as worrying. It's all mental effort and activity at a time when it shouldn't be happening. Whatever it is that's on your mind, it's stopping you from sleeping and living your life the way you want to.

As a result of the ongoing or recurrent sleeplessness, you feel tired and unrefreshed the next day. You might find it difficult to focus and concentrate, you might experience fatigue, feel low and irritable and get easily upset if your partner says something seemingly innocent, like your hair looks different. The daytime consequences and correlates of insomnia are much the same as the ones we discussed in chapters 6 and 7. But instead of you restricting your sleep, as happens if you go to bed too late, this is an ongoing sleep disorder that *stops* you from sleeping. Clearly, the more frequent the problems and the longer the problems persist, the more severely your performance and mood become affected. I've had clients who changed jobs and went part-time while others stopped driving because they had sleep problems almost every night. Others don't go on holiday anymore because they feel they'll make everyone miserable and be a burden to their hosts for getting out of bed at night when they can't sleep. Does any of this resonate with you? How has insomnia impacted your life?

When reading about insomnia you might have noticed the terms chronic insomnia and short-term/transient insomnia. Short-term insomnia is when you've been experiencing sleeplessness symptoms for fewer than three months. If it persists for longer then it develops into chronic insomnia, which is considered a sleep disorder. In western countries, the prevalence of chronic insomnia *disorder* is believed to be 10 to 12 per cent of the population; if you include acute insomnia, then the prevalence is 30 per cent and perhaps even 50 per cent.

Insomnia is one of the most common of all sleep disorders, which is why I'm going into so much detail. There's also a huge economic burden that comes with it in the form of lost productivity and health care costs. Unfortunately, it's on the rise in *all* age groups, although older adults are more at risk due to the influences of additional illnesses or health issues they may have along with other age-related changes in sleep regulation. For women, the risk for developing insomnia is higher than for men (hormonal fluctuations and family responsibilities might play a role).

# Why can't I sleep?

Although there are some 'risk' or predisposing factors that make some of us more prone to insomnia, having any of these doesn't mean you'll definitely develop insomnia. Which brings me to the question you're probably most interested in: 'Why can't I sleep?'

There's no easy answer because, although you might not realize it, you're asking not one but three questions. First, you're asking about the cause of insomnia, the 'thing' that triggered it. Second, you want to know what keeps insomnia going, what fuels it. Third, you wonder why *you* can't sleep while the rest of the world can. But I'm sure you're also wondering if there's anything you can do to 'get rid' of your insomnia. I'll come to that later. Let's start with the question about causes.

Many of my clients know what caused their insomnia. For some it was the frequent travelling to work, for others it was becoming a parent. Some clients are able to pinpoint the exact day (or night, I should say) that it started, such as the night before an important exam. Others don't know; they think insomnia crept up on them over time and one night they 'suddenly' found themselves lying awake with their mind racing and their body tossing and turning. And then there are those who might have never been a good sleeper. As you can see, there are many different causes for insomnia and each has its own, unique and personal stories attached to it. But if we look in more detail, some common characteristics and similarities emerge between the people who come to see me and in their stories. There are a number of behavioural, physiological, psychological and environmental factors that interact and can trigger insomnia — think of them as the raw ingredients, if you like. In mid-1980s Arthur Spielman, a pioneer in sleep research, developed a neat model classifying them into predisposing, precipitating and perpetuating factors, also referred to as the 3 Ps. (By the way, some factors fall into more than one category.)

# Predisposing factors

Predisposing factors (also known as risk factors) are biopsychosocial characteristics that increase the likelihood for insomnia: genetics (family history), being female, age, living alone, socioeconomic status, a higher metabolic rate, an overactive stress system (the amygdala is included here), hyper-activity (physiologically and psychologically hyper-alert), worrying or ruminating excessively and the often cited racing mind are some common examples. Your lifestyle and how well your internal bedtime (set by your internal clock) matches your actual bedtime (and the time you actually try to fall asleep) are other risk factors which make you more susceptible. Medical and psychiatric comorbidities (comorbidities describes when two or more health issues exist alongside one another and can sometimes influence each other) can predispose you to insomnia, while for someone else they function as a trigger. It really depends on your specific situation.

- - - - - - - - - - - - - - - - - - - - - - - -

Insomnia is often linked to a psychiatric illness such as anxiety, schizophrenia and depression (more than 80 per cent of people with depression suffer from insomnia), or physical conditions including cardiovascular diseases, medication (or a change in medication) and pain, as well as substance abuse. Often the cause–effect relationship is not clear, while in some cases insomnia is caused by the already-existing condition. In other cases, insomnia precedes the condition, perhaps even increasing the risk of developing hypertension or anxiety disorders, for example.

Whether insomnia is the cause or effect, both insomnia and the comorbidity need to be treated as each can exacerbate the other condition!

- - - - - - - - - - - - - - - - - - - - - - - - -

# Precipitating factors

Also known as triggers, precipitating factors are acute stressful events that spark off insomnia. General worries and stress such as losing your job (or getting a promotion), relationship problems, a death, an illness or changes in medication, alcohol and caffeine consumption, repeated loud noise at night or becoming a parent can all cause sleeplessness. Distressing as well as positive, exciting events can trigger insomnia, although the latter do so less often. These stressors are usually short-term and once the situation is resolved and you have adjusted, insomnia passes and normal sleep can return.

However, in some cases sleeplessness persists and develops into chronic insomnia. Why? Well, you got a taste of what sleeplessness means for your everyday life and — understandably — didn't like it. So while you no longer worry about the actual stressor, you now worry about not sleeping and how it affects you. And that's when the vicious cycle of chronic insomnia starts and the perpetuating or maintaining factors come into force.

Initially, you experience poor sleep because of some acute stressor. Soon you begin to notice how unpleasant this lack of sleep is and how it affects you in your daily life. You then start to worry if the sleep problem will ever stop. Thoughts like, 'I don't like feeling like this!', 'I can't afford another sleepless night' or 'I really need to sleep tonight or I won't be able to do my job tomorrow' might cross your mind as you get into bed or when you wake up at 4 a.m. You toss and turn, struggling with this horrid wakefulness in the middle of the night while your partner is happily asleep.

After a few problematic nights, sleep is on your mind as you get ready for bed, when you get home and eventually even during the day. 'This isn't good' you say to yourself, while gloomily drinking your third cup of coffee in the late afternoon to keep that sticky tiredness at bay. And so you start to do many different things to get your sleep back under control. For many of my clients, the need to control the insomnia soon takes over their life but the sleeplessness and the anxiety about not sleeping persist and continue to reinforce each other. And so the vicious cycle continues.

# Perpetuating factors

Perpetuating factors (also known as reinforcers) are behavioural and psychological factors that fuel your insomnia. They're considered maladaptive, because although you do them to cope with the sleeplessness, they actually make it worse and keep it going. You might start to exercise more, give up coffee because you realize it isn't helping you, and stop going out to meet friends so you can go to bed earlier. So you stay in bed for far too long. Or you decide to delay your bedtime so that you'll be really, really tired and surely able to fall asleep. To keep yourself awake you search the internet on your phone or watch a movie on your tablet. Maybe you try drinking alcohol as a way to get to sleep but then ban it altogether, looking longingly at the glass of wine your partner enjoys on a Saturday evening.

For me, the most prominent and powerful reinforcing factor is the repetitive and often negative thinking as you go to bed or when you wake up in the middle of the night. You ruminate about how insomnia affected your mood during that day, or worry about your ability to concentrate tomorrow. You become unhappy, which fuels even more negative thinking. But there's also a level of anxiety that sets in with worrying about the future and the consequences of not sleeping. This activates your body's stress system, which quickly puts you in a state of hyper-arousal (your amygdala is doing its job), making it hard for you to get to sleep or get back to sleep. Your heart's pounding, your breathing rate increases, your body or shoulders start to tense and by now the all-too-familiar knot in your stomach is present. On top of all these bodily sensations, your mind's racing at 100 miles per hour. This is certainly not a pleasant experience and when you get into bed the next night you're thinking about the previous night (ruminating) and wondering if you'll experience the same thing tonight, and you start to feel a little anxious (worrying). Over time, you start to associate lying in bed with these thoughts and the two become linked. Just thinking about going to bed or getting into bed, or about waking up in the middle of the night, triggers these unpleasant thoughts and emotions, causing you to become hyper-aroused. Researchers call this 'conditioned bedtime arousal'.

## Breaking the cycle

The question is, how can you break this vicious cycle to allow peaceful sleep to return? It's the perpetuating factors that you can really do something about. After all, it's your behaviour, the way you respond to your insomnia and those unpleasant thoughts and emotions that fuel it.

Practising healthy sleep habits and trying to reduce life(style) stressors is one aspect of an effective treatment. Then there are psychological and behavioural therapies that can help you. Cognitive behavioural therapy (often referred to as CBT) is a widely used multicomponent therapy with proven results. It aims to change your sleep-disruptive thinking through evaluating or challenging your thoughts. A newer therapy called Acceptance and Commitment Therapy (ACT) builds upon CBT and is informed by mindfulness; here you notice your unpleasant, negative thoughts and emotions and then accept them as they are. Using so-called defusion techniques, you learn to observe and step back from what's showing up in your mind and body. I now use ACT to help insomnia sufferers overcome their sleep problems.

Pharmacological treatment is another option, although for me this is more of a short-term rather than a long-term solution.

Taking sleeping pills can help you to break a cycle, but if insomnia becomes chronic I recommend going down the non-pharmacological treatment path. If you are taking them long-term, you run the risk of developing a drug tolerance, and may therefore need to increase the dosage as well as becoming addicted to the sleep medication.

# 10.

# HYPERSOMNIAS

Hypersomnias are a group of sleep disorders where, although you've had adequate sleep and perhaps slept for more than ten hours, you struggle to stay awake during the day and feel tired and unrefreshed, experiencing excessive daytime sleepiness (EDS). Because you're so tired, you sometimes fall asleep in the most inconvenient situations (having micro-sleeps or sleep attacks), which can have serious implications.

I'll introduce you to the most common or best-known hypersomnia disorders and their symptoms. Should you suspect that you or someone close to you might suffer from any of these, please consult your GP or sleep specialist. Please be aware that EDS or excessive sleeping can also be a symptom of other conditions including sleep apnoea, depression, substance abuse or multiple sclerosis.

## Narcolepsy

Narcolepsy is the most common hypersomnia disorder. The main symptom is feeling excessively tired during the day and struggling to stay awake. In addition, there are three other frequent symptoms you might experience, which I'll explain in further detail over the next few pages: sleep paralysis, hypnagogic hallucinations and cataplexy. Whether or not you experience cataplexy determines if you are suffering from narcolepsy type 1 (65 to 75 per cent of narcoleptics fall into this category) or narcolepsy type 2. Please be aware that these symptoms can also be related to other sleep disorders.

## EDS

If you suffer from narcolepsy you'll experience a higher than normal level of daytime sleepiness, or EDS. You can find it difficult to concentrate and remember things, and as the onset of narcolepsy occurs in your teens and twenties, this can have serious implications for your education, as well as your work life, personal life and social life. In its most severe form, narcolepsy can cause you to involuntarily doze off in the middle of a conversation or while driving (with severe consequences for your health and that of others). But while the feeling itself is no different to feeling sleepy after an entire night without sleep, the difference with narcolepsy is that you *did* sleep the previous night.

## Sleep paralysis

Some narcoleptics experience partial or total skeletal muscle paralysis at sleep onset or upon awakening. Normally, muscle paralysis occurs only during REM sleep and it takes a healthy sleeper over an hour to enter the first REM episode. When you're a narcoleptic, though, you enter REM much sooner, virtually as you are falling asleep. In a way, sleep paralysis is probably nothing other than the normal REM sleep paralysis intruding into your wakefulness or another sleep stage. For many people, this temporary inability to move is quite a frightening experience which can last for around a minute. I'll talk more about sleep paralysis when discussing parasomnias.

## Hallucinations

Sleep paralysis is often accompanied by hypnagogic hallucinations (which occur at the onset of sleep) and hypnopompic hallucinations (which occur during the process of waking up). These dream-like experiences are very intense, vivid, visually complex hallucinations, which is why they feel so real. Sometimes hallucinations may involve other senses, too. You might sense the presence of someone or something else with you in the room or even sitting on your chest. This leads to fear and dread and it can take a little while to disentangle yourself from these intense feelings.

Sleep hallucinations are another symptom of REM sleep intruding into wakefulness. Note that you might experience sleep paralysis and hypnagogic/hypnopompic hallucinations for other reasons; extreme sleep deprivation, for example, can also cause these sensations.

## Cataplexy

A cataplectic attack is a brief episode of muscle weakness that builds up over a few seconds and lasts up to several minutes. Cataplexy is similar to REM paralysis but unique to narcolepsy type 1. The feeling of muscle weakness can range from rather mild to a complete loss of body tone resulting in a fall to the ground. However, most episodes are less severe and the weakness only tends to affect the face, neck, arms or legs muscles. You might find that your speech slurs or your knees buckle.

An episode of cataplexy isn't the same as having a seizure or falling asleep — you don't lose consciousness during a cataplectic attack. It's usually triggered by strong emotions, more often positive rather than negative ones. Watching a comedy on TV, for example, can provoke an episode of cataplexy. Those people who experience episodes of cataplexy more often, or even lifelong, often learn what situations provoke a cataplectic attack and are thus able to control it to some level. Knowing what can trigger an episode helps sufferers to control it better.

– – – – – –

Unfortunately, there's still a lot to learn about what causes both narcolepsy type 1 and, especially, type 2. So far, it seems that some parts involved in the sleep–wake regulation in the brain aren't functioning the way they should, disrupting the normal cycle of wakefulness and sleep. What we do know is that narcolepsy affects women and men equally, and it's estimated that one in 2000 people is affected by the condition. (This incidence rate is similar to that of multiple sclerosis, so it's not uncommon.) Typically, the disorder starts in your late teens or early twenties and it can take some time until it's diagnosed correctly since narcolepsy is often misdiagnosed as depression, chronic fatigue or other medical and psychiatric conditions.

Although it's a lifelong condition with no cure it's possible to manage the condition and improve quality of life. There are several treatment options using medication to help to increase alertness and reduce cataplectic attacks, and lifestyle changes such as short, scheduled daytime naps to combat EDS, and of course sticking to regular bedtimes and wake-up times.

# Idiopathic hypersomnia

If you experience excessive daytime tiredness for more than three months and have no signs of narcolepsy or any other sleep disorder, you might be suffering from what's called idiopathic hypersomnia (IH) or hypersomnia of no known cause. Despite an adequate sleep duration, you feel unrefreshed and in fact find it quite difficult to overcome the effects of sleep inertia or sleep drunkenness when you wake up. You might even have slept for much longer than the recommended seven to nine hours, having slept for ten hours or more.

As with narcolepsy, IH usually starts in your mid to late teens or early twenties. In addition to age and genetics, gender might play a role. It seems that women are at greater risk than men — the prevalence is believed to be 50 in 1 million. Similar to narcolepsy, simply sleeping longer does not help to overcome IH. Many sufferers don't even feel refreshed after a long nap. There's no real cure for IH but, as with narcolepsy, the symptoms of IH can be managed through a combination of various treatment options as advised by a sleep specialist. By the way, IH is one of the few sleep disorders where a spontaneous remission can occur.

# Kleine-Levin syndrome

Sleeping Beauty isn't just the name of a fairytale, it's also the name of a hypersomnia disorder. Better known as the Kleine-Levin syndrome (KLS), sufferers recurrently sleep for twelve to 24 hours a day for a period of days, weeks or even months. The only reason they wake up is to eat and use the toilet — otherwise it's straight back to bed. Luckily, it's an extremely rare disorder, with a prevalence of perhaps 1 in 1 million. But, as with the other hypersomnias, it severely impacts your life, affecting young adolescents the most. What causes KLS is still unknown but it might be that infections, alcohol consumption and high levels of stress all contribute to the disorder. Currently, there's no real treatment for KLS but it often ends spontaneously after the age of around ten to fifteen.

## Behaviourally-induced insufficient sleep syndrome

If you regularly fail to get the amount of sleep that's right for you, you run the risk of developing behaviourally-induced insufficient sleep syndrome (BIISS), a widespread problem in our society these days. In contrast to other sleep disorders which have a medical cause, this is a voluntary sleep restriction; that is, your behaviour is responsible for the lack of sleep and the excessive daytime sleepiness or EDS.

There might be many reasons why we restrict our sleep: working shifts or long hours, socializing late in the evening or watching TV are just some of them. The key diagnostic criterion is that you are able to sleep longer if given the opportunity to do so. And that's also how you can 'treat' it — make sleep your priority and get more of it. This can be easier said than done, but have a think about what you can do. If you're a shift worker, talk to your boss about different work arrangements or nap opportunities at work. And engage your family and friends to ensure you get the sleep you need.

# 11.

# PARASOMNIAS

Parasomnia translates as 'something that arises or occurs alongside sleep' and that's exactly what happens in this group of common sleep disorders. Parasomnias involve a variety of unwanted physiological and behavioural events or experiences that can arise when you transition from one state to another, i.e. to and from wake (arousal), when transitioning back and forth between NREM and REM, or during a sleep state. When you have an episode of a parasomnia you might act or move in a way that's not typical for you and you might have abnormal dreams, perceptions and emotions. But although your behaviour makes perfect sense to *you*, you aren't conscious of what you're doing. For the people around you it might be a frightening, and in some rare cases dangerous, experience to observe because in reality your behaviour's just not appropriate. Anyone can experience parasomnias during their adult life but usually they're more common in children, simply because their brains are yet to fully mature.

The most commonly used classification system divides parasomnias into three main groups: NREM-related, REM-related and other parasomnias. I'll follow this system to look at some of the more frequent parasomnias.

# NREM-related parasomnias

This group of parasomnias is more likely to occur in the early part of the night when we experience more deep or slow-wave sleep. NREM-related parasomnias involve complex actions often resembling daytime behaviours and movements — except now you perform them at night. You might walk or talk, your eyes might be open but with a confused, 'glassy' look to them because you're 'absent' and completely unconscious of what you're doing. When you wake up you're disoriented and most *but not all* of the time you don't remember any of what has happened or the dream you just had. Sounds scary, right?

There are five NREM-related parasomnias in particular that I think are important to know more about. These are disorders of arousal; because parts of your brain have started to wake up while others are still asleep, you're partially asleep *and* partially awake. That doesn't mean there's anything wrong with you — you're not suffering from an underlying psychiatric disease. In an adult, sleep deprivation, different types of stress or medication can bring about episodes of NREM-related parasomnias. If episodes aren't too frequent or putting anyone in danger, treatment isn't needed to get your sleep back on track. Just ensure you're getting the sleep you personally need. I'll highlight the most pertinent points for each. If you are concerned, talk to a sleep specialist or your GP.

## Sleepwalking

Also called somnambulism, sleepwalking is when you sit up and get out of bed to walk around the house or even outside. Most of the activities you perform when sleepwalking will be mundane, such as talking or moving things around. But you might also try to climb out of the window or start to attack your partner, 'thinking' (or rather, dreaming) that someone's after you. It can be difficult to wake you up, but if woken you'll probably feel quite confused about what's going on. The best way to approach a sleepwalker is to speak to them very gently, slowly guiding them back to bed.

About 3 per cent of adults report sleepwalking, some experiencing episodes several times during the night. Others may only have a few episodes throughout their adult life. Episodes of sleepwalking are fairly normal for children. When I was about six years old, I managed to leave my parents' house, climb on the garden table and call for my granddad who lived in the house opposite. He used to sleep with an open window and when he heard my little voice calling, he spoke very softly as he approached and guided me safely back to my parents.

## Confusional arousal

Confusional arousal, also called sleep drunkenness, is when you behave in a confused and disorientated manner, shouting and thrashing about in bed. For one reason or another your sleep has been disrupted (maybe you have a cold or someone woke you up), and you seem to be awake but because you've just come out of deep sleep you struggle to understand what's going on around you. This state can last from a few minutes to a few hours, and it'll be hard to calm you during an episode because you're not fully awake. However, once the episode's over you might briefly wake up and then calmly go back to sleep.

## Sleep sex

Also known as sexsomnia, this is a disorder where you initiate sexual activity while still asleep. This is different from having an erotic dream, where you're paralysed (due to REM sleep paralysis) at that stage. Sleep sex can have severe interpersonal or even criminal implications.

## Night terrors

Night terrors (also called sleep terrors or *pavor nocturnes*) are frightening experiences (dreams) of profound panic while asleep. You wake up with a loud, spine-chilling scream, your heart's pounding and you're gasping for air. In some cases, you might be thrashing about or you may bolt out of bed and run around the house. Similar to confusional arousal, you're not fully awake when you experience an episode of night or sleep terror and trying to soothe you won't work. Night terrors usually last up to a few minutes, and because they happen in the first part of the night you can easily distinguish them from nightmares, which tend to happen more often during REM sleep.

Approximately 2 per cent of adults report night terrors. If episodes of night terrors are rare you do not need to seek treatment, but if you are concerned talk to a sleep specialist. It's also important to make the environment safe to protect yourself from injury.

## Sleep-related eating disorder (SRED)

This is another good example of a partial arousal from NREM sleep where you get out of bed to perform a daily activity — in this case, eating. But because you have no conscious awareness, your eating behaviour is fast, sloppy and out of control, and you go for high-calorie food and, let's say, peculiar combinations (e.g. coffee grounds or buttered cigarettes) while staying clear of healthy foods like fruit or vegetables. Typically, you can have one of these compulsive binge-eating and drinking episodes a night, although some sufferers will come back to the kitchen several times a night. The danger lies not only in overeating and weight gain but also in eating inedible substances such as detergents or uncooked foods (e.g. raw meat).

It seems that up to 5 per cent of the general population suffer from SRED, which is similar to the parasomnias we have discussed so far. However, women are two to four times more likely to be affected than men.

# REM-related parasomnias

REM-related parasomnias typically emerge during the second half of your sleep period. Contrary to NREM parasomnias, during which you're partially asleep and partially awake, you're asleep and able to move. When you awake from a REM-sleep parasomnia you're usually alert and able to recall your dream. Let me introduce you to some of the classic and sometimes peculiar REM parasomnias in the following sections.

## REM sleep behavioural disorder (RBD)

During REM sleep behavioural disorder (RBD) you act out your vivid and often aggressive dreams. You might kick, fight and shout or you might sing and laugh while sleeping. The paralysis or muscle atonia you usually experience during REM sleep is weakened, allowing you to move. It's also possible to wake you up during an episode of RBD and usually you can recall your dream, which again is different to NREM-related parasomnias.

Enacting your violent dreams does not mean you are more aggressive than others, though. It is worth bearing in mind that you are not conscious of your behaviour — you are in a dream experiencing something threatening against which you are defending yourself. Your aggressive behaviour is not aimed at your bedfellow — but of course there is a risk of injuring yourself or your partner!

The frequency of episodes of RBD varies among sufferers; for some it happens just a few nights per week, while for others it can happen every 90 minutes (remember the sleep cycles?). RBD tends to affect men over the age of 50 and its prevalence in the general population is less than 1 per cent. There seems to be an association between long-term RBD and some neurodegenerative disorders. Alcohol withdrawal and certain medications can acutely cause RDB but this is only short-term and will pass once things have normalized. Severe cases of RDB can be treated with medication, and your GP or sleep specialist will be able to advise you on the best pharmacological strategy. I would recommend making your sleep environment safe by removing sharp objects and providing additional padding to furniture to protect you from injuries. And as with everything, make sleep a priority and avoid sleep deprivation.

## Sleep paralysis

Sleep paralysis is the inability to move either when you're falling asleep or upon awakening. Sleep paralysis is a typical feature of REM sleep, but if it recurrently occurs outside of REM sleep or with narcolepsy it's considered a sleep disorder. I mentioned it as a symptom of narcolepsy but it can also occur on its own, which is what I am talking about here. What seems to happen is that the normal REM muscle atonia intrudes into wakefulness and you're unable to talk or move for a few seconds or minutes.

For many people, this temporary inability to move is a frightening experience because you're fully aware that it's happening. You might feel that something or someone is present in the room, weighing down on your chest and making breathing difficult. A good friend of mine once told me about his experience, which was exactly that. He woke up in the early morning hours and knew that something was present in the room, opposite his bed. He cried out, 'There's a demon high up in the right-hand corner!' He was scared and wanted to hide, but found himself unable to move. He said it felt as if his eyes were wide open with panic and fear at not being able to move. His cry woke up his wife. She knew nothing was there and that he was experiencing an episode of sleep paralysis, so she laid her hand on his arm to gently wake him up fully and soon the fear dissipated.

- - - - - - - - - - - - - - - - - - - - - -

*The Nightmare* by Henry Fuseli (1781) is one of the best-known paintings that captures the feeling my friend and so many others describe. Descriptions of sleep paralysis go back centuries, and interestingly almost all cultures depict it as something supernatural and evil. I know it can feel very real but I can assure you that what you are experiencing is a hallucination and nothing else.

- - - - - - - - - - - - - - - - - - - - - -

The experience of sleep paralysis isn't uncommon. For approximately 8 per cent of adults this is a recurrent condition, and about one-third of all adults will experience at least one episode during their life. Sleep deprivation and other poor sleep health habits, stress and high consumption of alcohol are among the usual suspects when looking for triggers for sleep paralysis. There also seems to be a genetic component to it; if a relative has it you're more likely than the average person to also get it. Treatment will depend on what causes your sleep paralysis; usually it's a combination of pharmacological and behavioural strategies.

## Nightmares

Nightmares arise mainly during REM sleep but in rare cases they can also occur during NREM sleep. Most of us will experience nightmares at some point during our life and this is absolutely normal. However, if nightmares occur frequently and recurrently, and affect your daytime mood and cognition because you don't get restful sleep, then they're considered a sleep disorder.

Regardless of their frequency, nightmares are dreams with intense negative emotion. Many people who have nightmares wake up during the night frightened by what they've just dreamt about. Usually they're able to recall the dream and continue to experience the feelings of, for example, anxiety, embarrassment or anger elicited by the nightmare. Being in a state of fear or anger, you might then not be able to go back to sleep. Sometimes you might even be too scared to go to bed the following night.

Different physiological and psychological factors can cause both occasional and recurrent nightmares. About 4 per cent of adults suffer from what is termed nightmare disorder, where nightmares are persistent and recurrent. Being ill, sleeping in an uncomfortable position or taking certain medications can cause nightmares. But they might also be a pernicious effect of everyday life stress, anxiety or psychiatric disorders such post-traumatic stress disorder (PTSD). If you suffer from nightmares, talk to your GP or a sleep specialist. Treatment for nightmares varies depending on the underlying cause. Apart from relaxation techniques to calm your anxiety or changes in medication, image rehearsal therapy (IRT) can be helpful. Here, you recall your dream as it was and then create a modified version of it, which you rehearse daily over the next couple of weeks. That way, you confront yourself with your anxiety and slowly learn to cope with and overcome it.

## HELPFUL HINT

If you experience nightmarish dreams but aren't sure whether you're experiencing nightmares or sleep terrors, pay attention to the timing and whether you can recall the content of the dream. Sleep terrors occur in NREM sleep and *usually* aren't remembered, whereas nightmares are well-remembered bad dreams that arise typically during REM sleep (see Figure 2 on p. 19 to remind yourself when REM sleep typically occurs throughout the night).

## Other parasomnias

As you might expect from the title, the category 'Other parasomnias' is a diverse group of parasomnias. Most of these disorders are benign in nature, and in most cases they don't need treatment. The best way to respond to them is to reassign your sleep the priority it deserves and explore ways to lessen any stress or emotional distress you're experiencing so that restful sleep can return.

## Sleep hallucinations

Sleep hallucinations are vivid imaginations perceived just as you're about to fall asleep or when you're waking up. We discussed them as a symptom of narcolepsy (see p. 151) so I won't go into too much detail here. Sleep hallucinations range from simple shadowy images to complex sensory imaginations. You may have had cenesthopathic feelings, i.e. abnormal sensations such as a light touching, a body part changing location, feelings of levitation or 'out of body' (extracorporeal) experiences.

Sleep hallucinations are very common, especially among the younger population. You might experience them on their own or together with other sleep disorders such as sleep paralysis or sleepwalking, for example. As frightening as they can be, they're not real — they're dream-like experiences and will disappear after a few minutes. Note that I say *dream-like* and not dreams. Sleep hallucinations arise when the brain misinterprets sensory information at the transition from one state to another, whereas dreams occur when you're actually asleep.

## Sleeptalking

Sleeptalking, or somniloquy, can occur in any sleep stage, either on its own or alongside another sleep disorder such as sleepwalking or RBD, for example. Sleeptalking is a phenomenon during which you don't move but you talk, sometimes quite loudly. What you talk about can vary: sometimes it might be just a word, at other times a whole story. Usually it's completely harmless but it might possibly be a bit rude and offensive to the listener.

Somniloquy is a common parasomnia. About 5 per cent of adults talk in their sleep. It's nothing to worry about and probably caused by emotional stress and lack of sleep.

## Sleep enuresis

Sleep enuresis, or bedwetting, is the involuntary voiding of urine during your sleep. It often results from a combination of factors affecting your bladder, such as volume or activity. It could be down to substantially reduced levels of vasopressin, an antidiuretic hormone that normally increases overnight to reduce the amount of urine in your bladder. Or it may be a difficulty with waking up to go to the toilet. Behavioural therapy and medication are effective in managing sleep enuresis.

## Exploding head syndrome

Exploding head syndrome (EHS) is characterized by an imagined loud noise or sense of explosion in your head while you are falling asleep or during the night, which wakes you up abruptly. People who experience EHS have described the noise as cymbals clashing, a bomb explosion or a beep. You don't feel confused when you wake up, and you can easily and clearly recall what just happened. Sometimes the sound is accompanied by a flash of light in front of your eyes, your body jerks and you feel distressed or frightened when you wake up. However, typically there's no pain associated with this rather violent noise sensation, which is what sets EHS and headaches apart. An episode of EHS doesn't last long; a few seconds and then it's over.

You may experience an attack very rarely, when extremely stressed. But some people can have several attacks a night, which is more than disturbing to their sleep.

## HELPFUL HINT

When you're dealing with someone who suffers from a sleep disorder, and a parasomnia in particular, remember that they're asleep when they behave abnormally. They might appear to be awake but they're not (or at most they're only partially awake). They're in a dream or dream-like experience, which can often cause them to experience extreme feelings of fear and anxiety. Naturally, they'll want to escape the situation or defend themselves against what, in the dream, is threatening their life. The best way to respond is to stay calm, and then wait until the next morning to discuss what happened.

Consult a sleep specialist if you or a loved one suffers from parasomnias, and discuss what measures to take to better manage parasomnias and the safety of yourself and others.

# 12.

# CIRCADIAN RHYTHM SLEEP-WAKE DISORDER

In circadian rhythm sleep–wake disorder (CRSWD) your internal sleep times are misaligned with the environment. You struggle to initiate or maintain sleep at times you (or your social environment) would like to. If you manage to sleep, it's likely to be of poor quality and/or too short. And we already know what follows on from that — a reduced quality of life.

In the following pages I'll briefly highlight the most pertinent points of the different CRSWDs and how they can affect not only your performance and concentration, but also your overall quality of life. I've already discussed jet lag in Chapter 2 so I won't mention it here.

## Shift work disorder

Shift work disorder (SWD) occurs when you — or rather, your internal clock — finds it hard to adjust to working at night and being asleep during the day. In a way, it looks like insomnia: a struggle to sleep during the day and excessive tiredness while on night shift. Most of us would initially find it difficult to adapt to this new routine, but after some time it usually becomes easier. But for up to 30 per cent of night-shift workers (and perhaps a little over 20 per cent of rotating shift workers) these problems persist and seriously affect their health and ability to function at work and at home.

There's no one-size-fits-all approach to helping shift workers sleep better. Many strategies are tailored to the individual and the organization. I have spent a lot of time talking to shift workers, learning about the nature of their work and developing such strategies to improve sleep, performance and safety. These might include educating people on sleep and also on fatigue (important in the context of shift work), or making changes to the sleep environment and protecting the daytime sleep period, restructuring breaks or looking at the shift schedules using a computer model, to name but a few. While these strategies help to manage the risk of fatigue, they of course won't make the underlying problem — namely that of having trouble sleeping in the daytime — go away.

## Delayed sleep phase disorder

Delayed sleep phase disorder (DSPD) is characterized by a *constant* delay of your internal clock. Your clock runs slower and your intrinsically preferred sleep times are much later than conventional sleep times. The duration and quality of your sleep are both 'normal' — it's simply that you want to go to sleep at a much later time than most people, perhaps between 2 a.m. and 6 a.m. That's three to six hours later than is conventional. To use the common bird analogy, you're a proper night owl!

The problem only arises when you try to go to bed at an earlier time than your clock wants you to, usually because you have to be up at a certain time the next day. You find it difficult to fall asleep, toss and turn and might even think you have sleep onset insomnia. When you finally fall asleep it's almost time to get up again. Needless to say, you feel tired for most if not all of the following day. But as soon as you're free to choose your sleep times you don't suffer any adverse symptoms or adverse consequences to your daily life. DPSD is a good example of a mismatch between social obligations (driven by social clocks) and your personal/intrinsic sleep pattern (driven by your internal clock) and how it can affect not only your emotional and physical health and wellbeing but also your performance.

We know how a lack of sleep (quality and/or duration) can affect your daytime performance and mood. This in turn can have major implications for your career and your relationships, because you'll continue to face the same problems unless you're free to choose your sleep (and work) times. Adolescents are the most likely to experience DSPD (with around 7 to 16 per cent of teenagers experiencing it) and might suffer the worst long-term consequences, with their school grades being affected and their future potentially compromised. But it doesn't stop there. Adolescents (and adults) with DSPD are also more likely to suffer from symptoms of anxiety and depression. They're also more likely to engage in so-called negative health behaviours such as smoking and consuming alcohol and caffeine in large quantities.

Why are adolescents more affected than adults? It's because of the natural biological delay of the internal clock that occurs during teenage years. Teenagers aren't just lazy when they won't get out of bed to go to school; it really is too early for them. However, not every teenager will suffer from the disorder. The majority are likely to experience a milder form with less severe symptoms. Also, using LED devices and watching TV in the evening doesn't help with a naturally delayed internal clock. It might be worth discussing this with your children.

Melatonin and light therapy have been shown to be effective strategies for treating DSPD. Talk to your sleep specialist for more guidance so that both of these treatments are timed to your (or your child's) specific circumstances.

# Advanced sleep phase disorder

Advanced sleep phase disorder (ASPD) is the exact opposite of DSPD. It is caused by a *constant* advance of your internal clock. It runs faster and your intrinsic sleep times are much earlier than conventional sleep times. Do you find it hard to stay up until more conventional bedtimes like 10 p.m. or 11 p.m.? Do you prefer to go to bed between 6 p.m. and 9 p.m., or even earlier? And do you then wake up early, at some time between 2 a.m. and 5 a.m.? If your answer's yes, then it's likely you're suffering from ASPD. Your sleep duration and quality are normal for your age, it's simply that you want to sleep at a much earlier time (three to six hours earlier than is conventional) and so wake up earlier — to hear the larks sing!

But, unlike DSPD and because of how our society works, ASPD has a much less severe effect on your performance and career. Your personal and social life might be somewhat affected, though, because you need to go to bed much earlier than most of your friends. As annoying as it might be, it's vital you go to sleep when your internal clock tells you to. Otherwise you shorten your sleep, because your clock will still wake you up at an early time and your daytime performance and mood will suffer. That's when you're likely to reach for the additional cup of coffee or other stimulant late in the day or evening.

There's a strong genetic link in ASPD, though it is much less common than DSPD; it occurs in only about 1 per cent of middle-aged adults, for example. However, the older you get the more likely you are to develop ASPD, plus there are also environmental factors and social and work pressures that might contribute to its development.

If you feel your life becomes affected by this disorder, include behavioural and light therapies. Use a light box in the evening and gradually delay your bedtime until you get to a time that you want to go to bed. Then stick to this new sleep–wake schedule as best as you can.

## Non-24 hour sleep–wake disorder

In non-24 hour sleep–wake disorder (Non-24) your internal clock won't entrain to the external light–dark cycle. Instead, it runs according to its own rhythm. Your clock's rhythm is longer than 24 hours, because it delays from day to day, whereas the external world runs according to a 24-hour cycle.

What does that mean for you? Well, you alternate between phases of disturbed sleep and excessive daytime tiredness, and phases of good sleep (coinciding with the external night-time). Over the course of twelve months your sleep–wake schedule will be out of sync with the rest of the world for most of the time. Because of your ever-changing sleep–wake patterns you might find it difficult to hold down a job and have a 'normal' family and social life. Insomnia-like symptoms and daytime tiredness are the other most frequently reported complaints when you suffer from Non-24.

Non-24 is most common in blind people with no light perception. That's because there's no entraining signal for the internal clock to anchor itself to. The reason it occurs in sighted people is currently unknown. It might be because of an extremely slow internal clock with a long cycle length (as in DSPD), a weakened response to light or environmental conditions (such as spending too much time in a dimly light environment) or psychiatric illness. Or it might be the result of your lifestyle, such as having an unstructured sleep–wake schedule and unhealthy sleep habits.

Overall, Non-24 is the rarest of the circadian rhythm sleep–wake disorder. The disorder is in itself harmless. And if you're able to follow your own sleep–wake rhythm, your sleep duration is the same as in normal sleepers of your age. Still, how can we help people with Non-24? Give your day a structure, get a routine. Have regular mealtimes and social engagements. Exercise at regular times, on the same days of the week. And above all, have a regular light exposure pattern with a focus on exposure to morning light. Of course, that won't help blind people with no light perception. Apart from timed melatonin administration, there's a new drug that has been shown to help entrain the internal clock to a 24-hour rhythm in totally blind people, enhancing their quality of life.

# Irregular sleep–wake rhythm disorder

With irregular sleep–wake rhythm disorder (ISWRD) the sleep–wake pattern is completely disorganized and there's no rhythm to it. You sleep at multiple times across the 24-hour day. Sometimes you might nap; at other times you might sleep for four hours. The problem is that your night-time sleep becomes fragmented and you won't get the amount of deep sleep you need to feel refreshed and energetic the next day. But if you add up the sleep you get over 24 hours, it's the same duration as for a normal sleeper your age.

This is similar to what we saw with Non-24. Sleep-maintenance insomnia and excessive daytime tiredness are the most common complaints of people who suffer with ISWRD. Having an irregular sleep–wake schedule makes it very difficult to keep a job and have a normal social and family life. As a consequence, you might feel depressed and isolated from everyone.

This disorder is the one circadian rhythm sleep–wake disorder that's primarily caused by a dysfunctional internal clock. A lack of light and the absence of a stable social schedule are other factors that can contribute to ISWRD, especially in people with a weak internal clock. This highlights how important it is for all of us to seek the sun on a daily basis and to have a regular, yet not fixed, lifestyle.

What can you do to treat your ISWRD? Get active and get a routine (this is similar to treating Non-24). Expose yourself to bright light in the mornings for about two hours. Make sure you put in place a healthy sleep habits regime. At night, keep it dark and quiet. And maybe take melatonin to help to reduce night-time awakenings and get your clock back on track.

## To sum up

Instead of summarizing the main points for each sleep disorder, I want to highlight a few common factors or causes, and treatment options.

Apart from genetic disposition, psychiatric and medical conditions, your lifestyle and behaviour play a big role in the development of multiple sleep disorders. Lack of sleep and high levels of stress — in particular emotional stress — are other common causes for sleep disorders. And once sleep is disturbed the chance of developing another sleep disorder or a medical condition increases.

One thing that's directly under your control is your lifestyle and behaviour. Making sleep a priority by adhering to healthy sleep habits, and reducing emotional distress are common and effective strategies to alleviate and manage or even resolve many sleep disorders. See the next section of the book for more details on good sleep habits. I think your health and that of your partner is worth it, don't you?

# part 4

# WEAVING HEALTHY SLEEP HABITS INTO YOUR LIFE

- - - - - - - - - - - -

I wake to sleep. I take my waking slow.

Theodore Roethke, 1953

Has it ever crossed your mind why we don't sleep enough? Sleep is essential for both our mind and body; nothing can function optimally without it. It's a precious commodity. So why is it that we don't better look after what's so important for our health and wellbeing? Sleep is nature's way of protecting us and allowing us to nurture ourselves, so why don't we give it the priority it deserves?

There's a plethora of reasons. Rarely is it just one factor that stops us from going to bed when our clock wants us to, and seldom is it one single cause that keeps our mind engaged while lying in bed. More often than not, a combination of different factors comes together in a way that results in us not sleeping enough or experiencing poor sleep. It's important to note that while some reasons are under our control, others just aren't. And the way all these factors and causes play out can be different for each one of us. Stress, work demands, family life, social engagements, lifestyle, light exposure, health, sleep disorders, and socio-economic status are the most common factors. They all can impact your sleep by willingly or unwillingly reducing the time you have for sleeping, or by keeping your mind busy and preventing you from falling or staying asleep. It goes beyond the scope of this book to make suggestions about how we as a society need to change, but change is needed. Lack of sleep is costing the economy billions of dollars in the form of lost productivity and health care costs. But more importantly, it's people's health and wellbeing that's at risk. Sleep needs to be held sacrosanct if everyone is to have a good quality of life.

In this section, I'll focus on those factors that are under your control, the ones you can work on directly. And the number one factor that underpins all others is your waking life, as it sets the scene for sleep the following night. What we do during our waking day, and how we do it, can affect if and how we'll sleep at night. And how we sleep at night can affect what we do, and how we do it, the next day. Of course, the same holds true for your emotions and mood. Sleep is a natural therapy.

Sleep and wake form a cycle: one follows as well as precedes the other. Therefore, each influences the other. To make this a positive influence, it's important to keep the boundaries clear between them. The beauty of this cycle is that we can start anywhere to make a change; we can intersect, if you like, at any point to improve sleep and thus daytime living. I propose you start by making sleep a priority and establish healthy sleep habits.

Healthy sleep habits shouldn't just address your evening or the time you are in bed. They should also include your daytime activities. The key is to identify healthy sleep habits tailored to what causes you to get less or poor sleep, and to your personal circumstances. Perhaps you are under a lot of stress because of work or family demands or you stay up late at night socializing with friends. Because reasons and circumstances vary between people and during different phases of your life, there's no one-size-fits-all approach, no one rigid list of healthy sleep habits to follow. *Religiously* trying to stick to each 'sleep commandment' all the time can do more harm than good to your sleep.

I want to share with you general healthy sleep habits to help you build *your* own scaffolding to support good sleep and minimize the occurrence of poor nights. Think of these as preventative measures. The more pieces you use for your scaffolding, the better protection it will provide. Similarly, the more often you practise these habits, the stronger your sleeping pattern will become and the more robust it will be against outliers such as a night of light or disturbed sleep. If the scaffolding analogy doesn't resonate with you, think of these sleep habits as a recipe for a meal. The more ingredients you add the better the meal, while at the same time if you don't have all of them you can still make the meal — albeit a slightly modified version.

One final thing: adopting healthy sleep habits doesn't mean you won't experience sleep problems. Some vaccines don't protect you completely against an infection. They do, however, lower the risk of getting the disease or lower the severity of the effects should you get the disease. And it's the same for following healthy sleep habits. They make your sleep more robust against sleep outliers.

# 13.

# A SCAFFOLDING FOR HEALTHY SLEEP

Healthy sleep habits start when you wake up in the morning. Remember, wake affects sleep and sleep affects wake. I've divided the general healthy sleep habits into different areas according to time of day and 'location' to make it easier for you to remember and implement them in your daily life.

You might find implementing these habits a struggle because of your current lifestyle, or maybe they simply don't resonate with you. Feel free to adapt them so they fit your individual circumstances. There's one thing I would ask you to keep in mind, though: are you making sleep a priority or are you letting other things take over? The more you appreciate sleep's importance for your health and wellbeing, the easier you'll find it to incorporate healthy sleep habits in your life naturally.

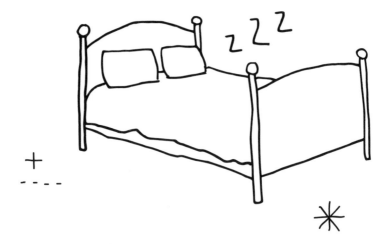

## Your sleep environment

### Make your bedroom comfortable

Spend some time in ensuring your bedroom is comfortable for you so that you feel able to 'breathe' and you will look forward to being in the room! Cosy is one thing, but too much clutter can keep your mind engaged or focused and drain your energy. So why not use the opportunity to tidy up and perhaps even redecorate a little to create a room that invites sleep? You could paint the room in a calming colour or get some furnishings with textures that call up a relaxed emotional state.

### Keep it dark

You don't have to have blackout curtains, because as much as we want to avoid light in the evening and at night, we want the light in the morning to help us wake up. Wearing an eye mask in the summer when the sun rises early or when you sleep in a room with no or very light curtains is okay, because the (light) stressor is actually present at the time we you want to minimize its effects. But try sleeping without it, or put it on only when it gets light, to avoid the risk of becoming dependent on it. And if the light from your electronic alarm clock bothers you, turn it away from the bed or get an old-fashioned clock.

## Keep it quiet

This can be tricky if you live near a busy road or somewhere like an airport, or if you have noisy neighbours. Using earplugs can be helpful in these cases because the (noise) stressor is actually present. But as a general rule, try to fall asleep without them and only use them as and when needed to avoid becoming dependent on them.

## Keep the room cool

Your body temperature naturally drops at night, which is important to get restful sleep. Sleeping in caves allowed for this, but well-insulated houses can sometimes make this difficult. Keep your bedroom temperature between 16 and 18°C (60–65°F). Fans, or if you have the luxury of air-conditioning, are great ways to help with the heat in the summer or for those living in warmer climates, but turn off all other electronic devices, as they give off heat. If you want to help your body stay cool, try putting a damp, wet towel over your forehead or on your legs. I know some people who have a cold shower while wearing lightweight clothing and then go to bed.

### The right bed and bedding for you

Get a bed and mattress that you feel comfortable in and that don't cause you any (extra) pain. Invest in good pillows and have summer and winter duvets (or alternate between woollen and cotton blankets) that accommodate the change in temperature from season to season.

# A healthy lifestyle: waking up

### Setting the scene

When you wake up, take a moment to acknowledge the sleep you got. I don't want you to get obsessive about the exact amount of sleep you had or fret about its quality. Simply reflect on your night and how your previous day influenced it. It's a bit like keeping a mental sleep diary.

Then take a moment to consider the day ahead of you, your to-do list and expectations. Plan moments in the day when you will step back and take a mini-mindfulness break, acknowledging what you're doing in that moment. Practising mindfulness regularly helps you to better regulate your emotions and reduce levels of stress. You slow down and develop a more balanced state of wellbeing — a pace and state that is more aligned with sleep.

### Keep your wake-up times regular

Make sure the time you wake up is regular — within a 30-minute time window. If you do stay up late one night on the weekend, get up the next day no later than 60 minutes after your normal wake-up

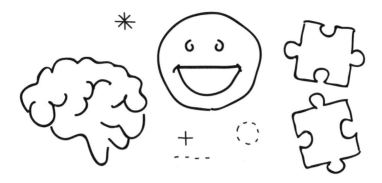

time. That way your internal clock won't get too confused and will find it easier to readjust to the natural 24-hour light/dark cycle.

### Getting out of bed

Once you're out of bed, open the curtains and let light in to help your body wake up and to ensure your internal clock stays synchronized or entrained to the solar day.

Air the bedroom and make your bed. Both behaviours can function as further signals that time in bed is over. Moreover, a made bed is so much more inviting to climb into in the evening!

If you practise meditation, now would be a good time to do it.

## A healthy lifestyle: during the day

### Sunlight

To help your internal clock keep aligned with the external day, spend time outside and let the melanopsin in your eyes 'soak up' as much sunlight as it can. (Just don't forget to put on sun protection for your skin!)

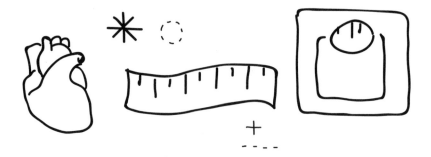

## Eating

Have a healthy diet and regular mealtimes. A healthy diet will reduce the risk of cardiovascular disease. Having regular mealtimes will help your internal clock to stay entrained to the 24-hour light/dark cycle.

## Stay hydrated

Remember, most foods also contain water so you don't have to have the often cited eight to ten glasses of water per day. However, when it comes to the evening time, reduce your intake of liquids to help minimize overnight toilet use. If you need to get up more than once during the night to use the bathroom, try to stop having liquids altogether one hour before bedtime. However, a sip of water as you go to bed or when you return from the bathroom is okay.

## Caffeine

If you drink coffee or other caffeinated beverages, do so moderately and strategically. Your alertness and cortisol levels rise naturally in the morning, so do you really need a coffee first thing every morning? See if you can wait until after 10 a.m. when cortisol levels have started to drop off.

And then there's the dip in alertness in the early afternoon, of course. You can have a coffee at this point to help you through the afternoon — but keep in mind that caffeine can stay in your system six to nine hours. As a rule of thumb, don't have more than a couple of cups of coffee per day and no later than 2.30 p.m. unless you need to be awake in the evening. Note, too, that most decaffeinated coffee or tea as well as certain foods still contain a small amount of caffeine. If you are sensitive to caffeine it might be best to avoid these, too.

## Dealing with stress

Set regular times for mini-breaks throughout the day to avoid or minimize the chances of getting stressed. Take 30 seconds to stop, become aware of the present and check in with your environment. Check in with how your body feels or what your breath does and then return to whatever you were doing. If you find you are stressed, then hopefully after a small break your mindset will have shifted a little and you'll see things more clearly.

## Daytime naps

Napping can help you to stay alert and boost your performance. Nap during the day if you feel you need to, but keep your nap to 30 minutes and no later than 3 p.m. so it doesn't interfere with night-time sleep.

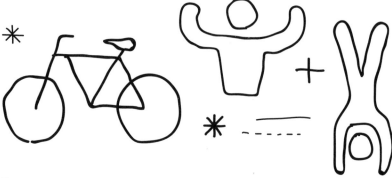

### Engage

Do one thing during the day that makes you smile to help maintain a positive frame of mind. This can be a simple, easy-to-do activity that you find engaging and meaningful — something that makes you feel good about yourself when you do it and which, when you reflect upon it at the end of the day, puts a smile on your face.

### Exercise

Lead an active lifestyle. Exercise regularly, but not within the last three hours before bedtime, otherwise it might negatively impact your ability to fall asleep by raising your body temperature too much. Exercise at this time might also provide too much extra stimulation and thus make falling asleep more difficult.

## A healthy lifestyle: the evening

### Your evening meal

Have a light and early dinner. This ensures your digestive system is not still working when it's time to sleep.

## Lighting

Lower the lights and minimize blue light exposure (from LED devices, including smartphones, tablets, laptops and close-range TVs). These act like mini-suns, increasing your alertness and affecting your internal clock by suppressing the release of melatonin. Moreover, the email or website content you're looking at is likely to provide further stimulation, keeping your mind engaged with daytime matters. So aim to turn them off three hours before bedtime.

## Alcohol and cigarettes

Moderate your alcohol intake or avoid it altogether. A glass of wine with your dinner or when you are out socializing is fine — for many, that's part of joyful living. But if you drink regularly in large amounts or use it as a sleeping aid, it can have adverse effects on your sleep, and health in general. (In Chapter 6 — see p. 107 — I discussed how alcohol can help you to get to sleep but disturbs the second half of your night-time slumber.)

If you smoke — and it's far better for your health and sleep if you don't — ensure you have your last cigarette at least two hours before going to bed. Nicotine is similar to caffeine in that it acts as a stimulant, making it harder to fall and stay asleep.

## Relax

Give yourself permission to feel tired. Wind down in the evening by doing something that's relaxing and nurturing. Spend time with your partner or family, read a book or magazine, watch TV (nothing too stimulating and not too late, though) or potter about. Perhaps listen to some music, not with the aim of getting you to sleep but because you like it and it helps you relax. Ultimately, it's about finding something that helps you to relax and allows you to have some quality 'me' time. (The term 'wind down' makes me think of little wind-up toys. Using that image, sleep is the wind-up phase, the daytime is the running phase and the evening is the final wind-down. Like the wind-up man, we have an inner clockwork. Living in tune with your inner clockwork, synchronized to the external day, will benefit your health and wellbeing.)

## Preparing for bed

If you like, take a warm bath 60 to 90 minutes before you go to bed. It will initially increase your body temperature but then help you to cool off much quicker.

Similarly, keep your feet warm. The body releases heat via the extremities but if you have cold feet or hands your veins will constrict, restricting the heat loss. Have a hot footbath and wear bed socks when needed.

If you fancy a little snack before bed, then eat something light. A blend of protein and slow-release carbohydrates is light, healthy and

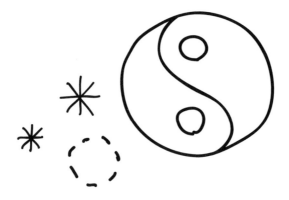

provides you with energy across the night. Try natural yoghurt with nuts and fruit, cereal with skimmed milk or crackers with a little cream cheese or organic peanut butter.

If you sweat a lot at night or suffer from hot flushes, try wearing lightweight sleepwear.

Set a regular bedtime, ideally in tune with your internal clock, and regularly go to bed within a 30-minute window of this time. Why not set an alarm to remind yourself?

Turn off your phone or put it on silent to minimize the risk of being disturbed during the night.

Pregnant women: sleep on your left side. Sleeping on your left maximizes the flow of blood and nutrients to your baby and uterus, and supports your kidneys to clear the body of waste fluids.

## Waking up overnight

If you wake up during the night and struggle to get back to sleep, stay in bed. Avoid using your phone, tablet or e-reader. Instead, try adopting an accepting attitude while allowing yourself to be awake rather than getting worked up and frustrated with the situation. I'll describe this approach in more detail in the next chapter.

- - - - - -

Some habits might be harder to implement than others at times depending on what's going on in your life. And that's okay; life happens and we need to adjust our behaviour. Scaffolding is built piece by piece, and some parts are more essential than others for it to stand. You need the floor pieces, for example, but you can do without the railing for a short while. Moreover, each building requires a slightly different set-up. You know being indoors all day and checking your work emails late at night isn't helpful for a good night's sleep but you can do it for a week if, for example, you're working on an international project. Or maybe you need to have a dark bedroom whereas your partner is able to sleep well in a room with sunlight coming in.

Build a set of sleep habits that makes sense to your life and that you're able to follow on most days and nights. But don't beat yourself up when you can't. Just try again the next day.

# 14

# DEALING WITH SLEEP ISSUES

This chapter outlines some natural ways to deal with issues such as a racing mind and the afternoon slump, as well as showing you how to identify the signs of tiredness.

## What to do when the mind starts racing

A racing mind that goes over the events of the day again and again, or worries about the next day, is the last thing you want when you are trying to fall asleep. And when you feel stressed, anxious or tense, sleep is nowhere to be seen. Naturally, you'll want to get rid of these thoughts, emotions and body sensations so you can fall asleep and get that peaceful sleep.

There are many different strategies on how to cope with these 'private events' (as research collectively refers to thoughts, emotions and body sensations) including cognitive behaviour therapy (CBT), relaxation and breathing techniques. Instead of reviewing each of them (you can find more information on these and other techniques online) I want to share with you a key element of the approach I teach all my clients and which they find very helpful.

The approach itself is called Acceptance and Commitment Therapy (ACT). I mentioned it on p. 147, and here's what I suggest you try. Observe the thoughts that go through your mind and the emotions and sensations that show up in your body. Rather than trying to get rid of them by distracting yourself or challenging the relevance of the thoughts, accept them. Allow them to come and go and to be just as they are without fighting them. It's almost like sitting in an armchair and noticing whoever is coming into the room. You don't talk or engage with them; you simply acknowledge them and then let them be. You don't get annoyed with yourself for thinking this way or feeling that way, you accept that what is there is there for now. You can practise this approach both during the day *and* if you wake up at night with worries or ruminations

If you continue to follow this approach, then over time you'll become less bothered by your thoughts and emotions, and will fall asleep much more quickly and will be able to return to sleep more quickly during the night if you wake up. Adopting an accepting attitude, rather than getting annoyed with yourself or frustrated with the situation, will help you save energy at night which you will then have for the next day.

I know this isn't easy when you first try it, because accepting something we don't like is a very different response to how we usually respond to a problem. I teach my clients mindfulness exercises to help them rebuild this capacity to just observe rather than judge. Maybe this is something you might find helpful, too. There's a lot of free content available online or — and this is what I would suggest — you can attend a mindfulness course in your local area. Gentle exercise and yoga during the day or early evening (not at night!) are nice accompaniments to a mindful way of living your life.

# If you need an afternoon alertness boost

Sometimes you're at work and feel tired but need to be awake and present for an afternoon meeting. Or perhaps you've had a run of poor nights, and getting through the day feels like a hard slog. What's the best way to get through the day?

## Caffeine

One option is to consume caffeine, for example coffee or black tea. Caffeine, a stimulant that keeps you awake, is the antagonist of adenosine. I discussed this in Chapter 1 but I think it's important to quickly recap. Adenosine is a biological indicator of your sleep pressure or sleep drive; the longer you're awake the higher the pressure and the more adenosine is in your brain attached to brain cells. Unless caffeine has been consumed. By binding to the same cells, caffeine prevents adenosine from binding and its 'sleepiness message' doesn't reach the cells (i.e. adenosine cannot signal the cells to slow down). Be aware that the levels of adenosine continue to increase while we stay awake, and the number of receptors on the brain cells also increases, which is why over time you need to drink more coffee to block these, too. Once the caffeine has finally been metabolized, all the accumulated adenosine binds to the free receptors, making us tired very quickly. In this way, caffeine is a bit of a cover-up, so to speak.

Caffeine also works as a stimulator. For example, it activates certain brain areas to trigger the secretion of cortisol and adrenaline by the adrenal glands. (I discussed cortisol in Chapter 5 when talking about sleep and diabetes.) Both hormones are involved in the fight or flight response and they increase your alertness and energy levels. You won't feel the effects of caffeine instantly; it takes about 20 minutes for caffeine to take effect. And, as mentioned, it takes about six to nine hours for the effects to completely wear off. So plan when to have your coffee so that it alerts you when you need it during the day (most likely in the early afternoon) but doesn't stop you from sleeping at night.

## Take a nap

Take a nap of no more than 30 minutes, and make sure it's no later than 3 p.m. Why these two restrictions? Firstly, to prevent you entering deep sleep — remember, it's easier to wake up from light sleep, which takes about 20 minutes (plus a few minutes to fall asleep). Secondly, regardless of when you do it, napping reduces your sleep pressure (the drive to sleep) while being awake increases it (see Chapter 1). If you nap too close to your normal bedtime (or nap too long, for that matter) you won't have enough time to achieve the right amount of sleep pressure so that you can go to sleep at your normal bedtime. Instead, you might stay up longer but because you still have to get up at the normal time in the morning you then don't sleep enough. (This is a good example of just how easy it is to experience sleep loss.)

## Daylight

Another way to help increase your alertness in the afternoon is to expose yourself to some strong light. Remember, from influencing the internal clock (see Chapter 2), light has strong alerting effects. Try to go outside even if it's an overcast day, as the natural light outdoors will be far brighter than the office light you usually spend your day in.

- - - - - -

The best booster of all is a combination of all three. Have a cup of coffee, nap for 20 to 30 minutes and then go for a brisk walk outside. And then interact with people to help improve your mood. As we know, your mood can suffer from a lack of sleep and make everything seem like a hard slog. Withdrawing from everyone might seem the best way forward, but it isn't. You'll just feel even more isolated. So do the opposite and chat with someone.

## How to spot tiredness

While (almost) everyone is aware of the dangers of drinking and driving, and thus follows the law to stay safe and keep others safe, the attitude towards not sleeping (enough) and driving is entirely different. The National Highway Safety Administration in the United States reports that 846 *fatal* driving accidents in 2014 were sleep related. Other research suggests that this is an underestimation and actual numbers are much higher. (This is probably similar for other countries, too.)

There are some warning signs that 'advertise' that you are tired or even fatigued, and that your performance is impaired. Some of these signs relate to cognitive performance, while others are physical signs, and again others relate to your emotional state.

In the table opposite I have listed the most important signs and symptoms and roughly order them by severity of tiredness (from top to bottom). Please note that the progress from being alert to being tired to being fatigued is a fluid one and these signs and symptoms do not all have to appear, and not always in this order.

Being aware of these symptoms of tiredness and fatigue is important in all areas in your life. They signal that you haven't had enough sleep or have been awake for too long. Eventually, the body will just take the sleep it needs and you start to experience micro-sleeps, brief moments where you unwillingly and unknowingly nod off. This is extremely dangerous when driving as you lose all awareness of the road and the ability to control your car. In a normal daily setting, such as at work or home, the risk to you and others is of course much lower, but nevertheless it would be embarrassing to just nod off in a conversation or meeting.

Knowing the different symptoms of fatigue can help you to perform better and be safer in both your professional and private life. And once you know the warning signs you are able to spot them in others and can hint to them that they would benefit from some extra zzzz's.

# How to spot tiredness and fatigue

| Severity | Physical | Cognitive | Emotional |
|---|---|---|---|
| | Yawning, rubbing eyes, fidgeting | Poor attention and communication, easily distracted (slips and lapses) | Quieter and more withdrawn |
| | Heavy eyelids, long blinks, staring blankly, lacking energy, droopy corners of the mouth, pale skin | Poor processing of information and memory | Lacking energy and motivation, low mood |
| | Head nodding, micro-sleeps | Poor situational awareness, poor decision-making and increased risk-taking | Irritability, aggression |

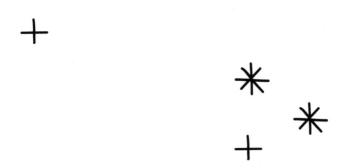
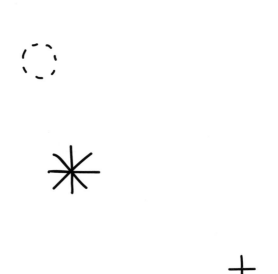

# PARTING WORDS

Together we've gone on a journey, a journey of sleep. The intention of this book has been to give you an understanding of why sleep is a top priority for everyone. By following this motto, you'll naturally find additional ways to best prepare for and then sleep at night.

In the first part of the book we looked at where and how sleep happens, and how the need to sleep changes across a 24-hour day. We looked at how light influences our sleep, and how it can help you to perform and feel better. Then we learnt about the gender difference in sleep and that there's more to discover on this specific topic. This last statement also holds true for dreams, another fascinating area we still know too little about.

The middle part of the book, and the one I consider the core, explored sleep and physical health, cognitive performance and emotional wellbeing. If sleep suffers, so will any, if not all, of these three pillars of healthy living. Turn it around and sleep becomes a vital protector of health and wellbeing. The next part examined sleep disorders and how to spot them. In the final part, I proposed a menu of healthy sleep habits for you. You don't need to follow them religiously, just in a way that makes sense to your lifestyle.

You might have read the book from start to finish or read the chapters in your own order. Whichever way, I hope you enjoyed the read. I hope it also satisfied your desire to learn more about sleep and helped you become excited to go to bed and nourish yourself tonight by sleeping.

Sleeping is, and always will be, simple. It's our waking life that makes it more complicated. Take a break and go outside to get natural sunlight. That can be the first step to disentangling yourself from a busy lifestyle and simultaneously preparing for your night-time sleep.

Warmly,
Katharina

# GLOSSARY

**Chronic insomnia disorder** *see* Insomnia

**Circadian clock** *see* Internal body clock

**Circadian rhythm sleep–wake disorders** A group of disorders resulting from a misalignment between internal and external time or changes to the internal time-keeping system (i.e. the internal, circadian clock).

**Cognition, cognitive performance** A range of mental processes or abilities which allow you to gain knowledge and comprehend it.

**Comorbidity** An additional disease or condition.

**Conditioned bedtime arousal** Occurs when sleep-related environments or situations (e.g. thinking of or getting into bed) are perceived as stressors, triggering hyper-arousal.

**Confusional arousal** A sleep disorder where the afflicted person behaves in a confused manner when sleep has been disrupted and they wake up from a deeper sleep stage.

**Delayed sleep phase disorder** A circadian rhythm sleep–wake disorder characterized by a *constant* delay of your internal clock.

**Exploding head syndrome (EHS)** A sleep disorder characterized by an imagined loud noise or sense of explosion in your head while you are falling asleep or during the night, which wakes you up abruptly.

**Ghrelin** A hormone produced by the stomach that stimulates your appetite.

**Hypersomnia**  Excessive sleepiness during the day interfering with day-to-day life.

**Hypertension**  Chronically high blood pressure.

**Hypnagogic hallucinations**  Hallucinations occurring when falling asleep.

**Hypnogram**  Graphical representation of the pattern of brainwaves during sleep.

**Hypnopompic hallucinations**  Hallucinations occurring when waking up from sleep.

**Idiopathic hypersomnia**  A type of hypersomnia without a known cause.

**Image rehearsal therapy (IRT)**  A technique to treat nightmare disorder involving recalling the original nightmare, modifying it and then rehearsing a new scenario.

**Insomnia**  A sleep disorder where the afflicted person has problems falling and/or staying asleep and/or waking up too early, and thus feels tired during the day.

**Internal body clock**  Located in the suprachismatic nuclei of the brain and provides a time measure to the body. Because it deviates slightly from the external 24-hour day, it is also called the circadian clock (from the Latin *circa*, meaning 'about' and *dies*, meaning 'day').

**Kleine-Levin syndrome**  A type of hypersomnia, the afflicted person will recurrently experience sleep episodes for more than eighteen hours a day.

**Leptin**  A hormone that signals the brain to inhibit food intake (among other functions).

**Lux**  The unit of measurement of light intensity levels.

**Melanopsin**  A novel photopigment sensitive to blue light.

**Melatonin** A hormone produced at night to signal to the body it is night-time.

**Micro-sleep** A brief, sudden, unintentional sleep episode.

**Narcolepsy** A hypersomnia disorder that causes excessive tiredness during the day and can cause the afflicted person to involuntarily fall sleep.

**Non-REM sleep (NREM) or non-rapid eye movement sleep** One of two sleep states.

**Night terrors (sleep terrors, *pavor nocturnes*)** A frightening experience while asleep from which the afflicted person often wakes up with a loud scream.

**Non-24 hour sleep–wake disorder (Non-24)** A circadian rhythm sleep–wake disorder where sleep times are misaligned with the external 24-hour day.

**Parasomnias** A group of sleep disorders involving unwanted physiological and behavioural events or experiences.

**Parasympathetic nervous system** The 'rest and digest' system of the autonomic nervous system.

**Polysomnography (PSG)** The measurement of sleep by placing electrodes on, for example, the skull and face.

**REM sleep or rapid eye movement sleep** One of two sleep states during which the body is paralyzed.

**Sexsomnia (sleep sex)** A sleep disorder where the afflicted person initiates sexual activity while asleep.

**Sleep architecture** The pattern or organization of NREM and REM sleep stages across the sleep period.

**Sleep drive (or sleep pressure)** The need to sleep that builds up with every hour of wakefulness.

**Sleep enuresis (bedwetting)** The involuntary voiding of urine during sleep.

**Sleep inertia**  A state of lower arousal upon waking up.

**Sleep-related breathing disorders**  A group of sleep disorders characterized by breathing problems.

**Sleep-related movement disorders**  A group of sleep disorders that includes involuntary movements during sleep (and sometimes before).

**Somnipathy**  The scientific terminology for a medical disorder of sleep patterns.

**Sympathetic nervous system**  The 'fight or flight' system of the autonomic nervous system.

**Vagus nerve**  Part of the parasympathetic system used to innervate most tissues and organs in the body.

# ACKNOWLEDGEMENTS

There are many people I would like to thank. My teachers and my clients for sharing their knowledge and experiences with me. Anouska Jones and Karen Gee from Exisle for their oversight, support and skilful editing. Peter Algate for his valuable suggestions on the manuscript. David Denni for his wonderful illustrations. I am indebted to my parents for their support and love. I am grateful to Alexander Barclay, my most sensible reader and critic, and my partner.

# REFERENCES

## 1. Sleep: the most frequent questions answered

Roenneberg, T. et al. 2003, 'Life between Clocks: Daily Temporal Patterns of Human Chronotypes', *Journal of Biological Rhythms,*18: pp. 80–90.

## 2. Light and sleep

Arendt, J. and Skene, D. 2005, 'Melatonin as a chronobiotic', *Sleep Medicine Reviews*, 9: pp. 25–39.

Chang, A.M. et al. 2014, 'Evening use of light-emitting e-readers negatively affects sleep, circadian timing, and next-morning alertness', *Proceedings of the National Academy of Sciences*, 112(4): pp. 1232–7.

Gooley, J. et al. 2001, 'Melanospin in cells of origin of the retinohypothalamic tract', *Nature Neuroscience*, 4(12): p. 1165.

Küller, R. et al. 2006, 'The impact of light and colour on psychological mood: a cross-cultural study of indoor work environments', *Ergonomics*, 49(14), pp. 1496–1507.

Provencio, I. et al. 2000, 'A Novel Human Opsin in the Inner Retina', *Journal of Neuroscience,* 2000, 20(2): pp. 600–5.

## 3. Sleep in women

Duffy, J.F. et al. 2011, 'Sex difference in the near-24-hour intrinsic period of the human circadian timing system', *Proceedings of the National Academy of Sciences*, 108(3): pp. 15602–8.

## 4. Dreaming

Hall, C.S. and Nordby, V. J. 1972, 'The individual and his dreams', New York: New American Library.

Mathes, J.M. and Schredl, M. 2013, 'Gender differences in dream content: Are they related to personality?' *International Journal of Dream Research*, vol. 6(2): pp. 104–9.

Nielsen, T. et al. 2004, 'Immediate and delayed incorporations of events into dreams: Further replication and implications for dream function', *Journal of Sleep Research*, 13: pp. 327–36.

Schredl, M. and Hofmann, F. 2003, 'Continuity between waking activities and dream activities', *Consciousness and Cognition*, 12: pp. 298–308.

## 5. Sleep and physical health

Axelsson, J. et al. 2010, 'Beauty sleep: experimental study on the perceived health and attractiveness of sleep deprived people', *British Medical Journal*, 341: c6614.

Dashti, H. et al. 2015, 'Short Sleep Duration and Dietary Intake: Epidemiologic Evidence, Mechanisms, and Health Implications', *Advances in Nutrition*, 6: pp. 648–59.

Eckel, R.H. et al. 2015, 'Morning Circadian Misalignment during Short Sleep Duration Impacts Insulin Sensitivity', *Current Biology*, 25(22): pp. 3004–3010.

Ishibashi, K. et al. 2007, 'Inhibition of Heart Rate Variability during Sleep in Humans by 6700 K Pre-sleep Light Exposure', *Journal of Physiological Anthropology*, 26(1): pp. 39–43.

Prather, A.A. et al. 2012, 'Sleep and antibody response to hepatitis B vaccination', *Sleep*; 35(8): pp. 1063–9.

St-Onge, M.-P. et al. 2016, 'Fiber and saturated fat are associated with sleep arousals and slow wave', *Journal of Clinical Sleep Medicine*, 12(1): pp. 19–24.

Wang, Y. et al. 2015, 'Relationship between Duration of Sleep and Hypertension in Adults: A Meta-Analysis', *Journal of Clinical Sleep Medicine*, 11(9): pp. 1047–56.

Wulff, K. et al. 2010, 'Sleep and circadian rhythm disruption in psychiatric and neurodegenerative disease', *Nature Reviews Neuroscience*, 11(8): pp. 589–99.

Xie, L. et al. 2013, 'Sleep drives metabolite clearance from the adult brain', *Science*, 342(6156): pp. 373–7.

## 6. Sleep well to perform well

Alhola, P. and Polo-Kantola, P. 2007, 'Sleep deprivation: Impact on cognitive performance', *Neuropsychiatric Disease and Treatment*, 3(5), pp. 553–67.

Dawson D. and Reid K. 1997, 'Fatigue, alcohol and performance impairment', *Nature*, 388(235): p. 235.

Hafner, M. et al. 2016, 'Why sleep matters — the economic costs of insufficient sleep: A cross-country comparative analysis', Santa Monica, CA: RAND Corporation. https://www.rand.org/pubs/research_reports/RR1791.html.

Van Dongen, H. et al. 2003, 'The cumulative cost of additional wakefulness: Dose-response effects on neurobehavioral functions and sleep physiology from chronic sleep restriction and total sleep deprivation', *Sleep*, 2: pp. 117–26.

## 7. Emotional wellbeing and sleep

Palmer, C.A. and Alfano, C.A. 2017, 'Sleep and emotion regulation: An organizing, integrative review', *Sleep Medicine Reviews*, 31: pp. 6–16.

Simon, E.B. et al. 2015, 'Losing neutrality: The neural basis of impaired emotional control without sleep', *Journal of Neuroscience*, 35(38): pp. 13194–205.

Thomsen, D.K. et al. 2003, 'Rumination: Relationship with negative mood and sleep quality', *Personality and Individual Differences*, 34(7): pp. 1293–1301.

Vandekerckhove, M. et al. 2011, 'The role of pre-sleep negative emotion in sleep physiology', *Psychophysiology*, 48(12): pp. 1738–44.

Vandekerckhove, M. et al. 2012, 'Experiential versus analytical emotion regulation and sleep: Breaking the link between negative events and sleep disturbance', *Emotion*, 12(6): pp. 1415–21.

## Part 3: When sleep goes wrong (chapters 8–12)

Clark, I. and Landolt, H.P. 2017, 'Coffee, caffeine, and sleep: A systematic review of epidemiological studies and randomized controlled trials', *Sleep Medicine Reviews*, 31: pp. 70–8.

Garvey, J. et al., 'Epidemiological aspects of obstructive sleep apnea', *Journal of Thoracic Disease*, 7(5); pp. 920–29.

Hayashi, M. and Hori, A.M. 2003, 'The alerting effects of caffeine, bright light and face washing after a short daytime nap', *Clinical Neurophysiology*, 114(12): pp. 2268–78.

Khan, Z. and Trotti, L.M. 2015, 'Central disorders of hypersomnolence: Focus on the Narcolepsies and Idiopathic Hypersomnia', *Chest*, 148(1): pp. 262–73.

Ong, J. et al. 2012, 'Improving Sleep with Mindfulness and Acceptance: A Metacognitive Model of Insomnia', *Behaviour Research Therapy*, 50(11): pp. 651–60.

Riemann, D. et al. 2015, 'The neurobiology, investigation, and treatment of chronic insomnia', *The Lancet Neurology*, 14(5): pp. 547–58.

Slama H, et al. 2015, 'Afternoon nap and bright light exposure improve cognitive flexibility post lunch', *Public Library of Science One*, 10(5): 30125359.

Spielman, A. et al. 1987, 'A behavioral perspective on insomnia treatment', *Psychiatric Clinics of North America*, 10(4): pp. 541–53.

Zhu, L. and Zee, P.C. 2012, 'Circadian rhythm sleep disorders', *Neurologic Clinics*, 30(4): pp. 1167–91.

# FURTHER READING

## Determining your circadian rhythm type

See the Center for Environmental Therapeutics website at https://www.cet.org/ and look for the 'self-assessments' link where you'll find the survey 'Your circadian rhythm type' that will help you determine your personal internal clock and therefore your best timing for light therapy.

## Munich Chronotype Questionnaire

The Munich Chronotype Questionnaire (MCTQ) was developed by a German research group led by Professor Till Roenneberg. You can complete the questionnaire online and get an instant response. Your data will also go into a larger data to help researchers find out more about when and how long people sleep around the globe. See https://www.thewep.org/documentations/mctq

## National Highway Safety Administration

For more information on how to combat tiredness or fatigue when driving, see https://www.nhtsa.gov/risky-driving/drowsy-driving#topic-scope-problem

## National Sleep Foundation

The National Sleep Foundation (NSF) is an independent non-profit organization dedicated to improving public health and safety through public understanding of sleep. It is 'the global voice for sleep health'. The NSF convened a panel of sleep experts and other experts to review the literature and develop recommended sleep duration for set age groups. In 2013, they conducted a sleep poll in the United States, Canada, Mexico, the United Kingdom, Germany and Japan. The results, published as the '2013 International Bedroom Poll', can be found here: https:// sleepfoundation.org/sites/default/files/RPT495a.pdf

## Sleep disorders

The classification system I used for the sleep disorders in Part 3 is based on the International Classification Sleep Disorders-3 (ICSD-3). If you would like to learn more about sleep disorders, here are some helpful websites.

**American Academy of Sleep Medicine**
www.sleepeducation.org/sleep-disorders-by-category

**National Sleep Foundation's e-book on sleep disorders**
sleepdisorders.sleepfoundation.org

**Snore Australia**
www.snoreaustralia.com.au/sleep-disorders.php

**The Stanford Center for Sleep Sciences and Medicine**
sleep.stanford.edu/sleep-disorders/

# INDEX

## A

Acceptance and Commitment Therapy (ACT) 147, 194
adenosine 15, 195
adolescents, DSPD 169–70
advanced sleep phase disorder (ASPD) 170–1
afternoon alertness boost 195–7
afternoon naps 30, 33, 35, 196
alcohol
  blood alcohol concentration 107
  effect on sleep 117, 189
alcohol withdrawal, RBD 160
alertness
  afternoon boost 195–7
  effect of light 46–7
  light as booster 49
  rhythm of 33–5, 34
Alzheimer's disease 96
amygdala
  diagram of brain 114
  overreactive 115
  response to stimuli 113
appetite hormones 83–4
arousal system 12–13
ASPD (advanced sleep phase disorder) 170–1
atherosclerosis 91
attention, ability to focus 112–14
autonomic nervous system 88

## B

beauty sleep 97
bedding 184
bedroom conditions 182–4
bedtime, preparing for 190–1
bedwetting 165, 205

behaviourally-induced insufficient sleep syndrome (BIISS) 154
blaming others 110–11
blind people, dreams 67
blood alcohol concentration (BAC) 107
blood pressure
  circadian rhythm 90–1
  magnesium 91
blue light 39–40, 47–8, 189
brain, sleeptime clean-out 95–6
breathing disorders, sleep-related 129, 131–6, 206

## C

caffeine 186–7, 195–6
cancer, cause of effect 95
cardiovascular diseases 92–3
cataplexy 151–2
CBT (cognitive behavioural therapy) 147
central sleep apnoea (CSA) 134–5
chronic insomnia disorder 141, 204
chronotype
  finding your own 25
  and sleep duration 31
cigarettes 189
circadian clock see internal body clock
circadian pacemaker see internal body clock
circadian rhythm sleep–wake disorder (CRSWD) 129, 167–73, 203
cognition
  performance 203
  role of sleep 78
cognitive behavioural therapy (CBT) 147
cognitive functions
  connection to sleep 99–101
  lack of sleep 113–14, 115–16
  in personal life 103–4
  role of body clock 104–5
  in workplace 102
comorbidities
  explained 203
  medical and psychiatric 143
conditioned bedtime arousal 203

confusional arousal 157, 203

continuous positive airway pressure (CPAP)
devices 134

coping strategies 119–20

cortisol 87

couch potato, dangers of being 83–6

creativity, from dreams 72

CRSWD (circadian rhythm sleep–wake
disorder) 129, 167–73, 203

CSA (central sleep apnoea) 134–5

cytokines 88, 92

**D**

darkness 48–9

daylight, help with alertness 197

daylight saving, effect of time change 93

daytime naps 187

decision-making, effect of fatigue 102–3

delayed sleep phase disorder (DSPD)
168–70, 203

diabetes 86–90

diet
effect on sleep stages 85–6
healthy habits 186

dim light melatonin onset (DLMO) 42–3

disasters, due to fatigue 102

DLMO (dim light melatonin onset) 42–3

dream functions, theories 66–7

dreams
common themes 73–4
continuity hypothesis of 73–4
creativity from 72
daytime activity 70
discontinuity 73
explained 65
men vs women 69–71
night terrors 158
REM sleep 21
REM sleep behavioural disorder 159–60
sleep stages 68
and waking life 68–9, 71–2

DSPD (delayed sleep phase disorder)
168–70, 203

**E**

earplugs 183

eating
healthy habits 186
late nights 82–3
reward system 85

EDS (excessive daytime sleepiness) 149,
150

EHS (exploding head syndrome) 165–6, 203

electronic devices
blue light 39–40
blue-light effect 48

emotional wellbeing
mood balance 109
role of sleep 78–9

emotions
ability to regulate 112–14
effect on sleep 118–20
processing 119–20

endothelium 92

energy, in the evening 35–6

engaged, staying 188

evening lifestyle 188–91

excessive daytime sleepiness (EDS) 149,
150

exercise 188

exploding head syndrome (EHS) 165–6, 203

eye mask 183

**F**

fatigue
signs of 197–9
widespread effects 102–3

friendships, effect of sleep loss 104

**G**

ghrelin 83–6, 203

grogginess, after waking 32–3

**H**

hallucinations 151

healthy lifestyle
during the day 185–8

the evening  188–91
waking up  184–5
heart attacks, peak time  93
heart health  92–3
heart rate
24-hour variability  92–3
cardiovascular diseases  93
hedonic drive  85
histamine  13
hot flushes  61–2
hydration  186
hypersomnia  129, 149, 204
hypertension  90, 204
hypnagogic hallucinations  151, 204
hypnic spasms  19
hypnogram  18, 19, 23, 204
hypnopompic hallucinations  151, 204

I
idiopathic hypersomnia (IH)  153, 204
IH (idiopathic hypersomnia)  153, 204
image rehearsal therapy (IRT)  204
immune system, sleep boost to  94–5
impulse control  110–11
indoor lighting  47
infectious diseases, short sleep  94
insomnia
breaking the cycle  147–8
causes  142–4
explained  204
impact of  141
perpetuating factors  146–7
precipitating factors  144–5
predisposing factors  143–4
three types  140
umbrella term  139–40
insomnia disorder  129
insulin resistance  86–7, 88
internal body clock
effect of light  38
effect of melatonin  41–3
expected light pattern  40–2
explained  16–18, 204

influence of light  51–2
signals sleep time  14
staying asleep  17–18
women  54–5
irregular sleep–wake rhythm disorder
(ISWRD)  172–3
IRT (image rehearsal therapy)  204
isolation, social  111–12
ISWRD (irregular sleep–wake rhythm
disorder)  172–3

J
jet lag  43–6
judgement, impaired  113–14

K
Kleine-Levin syndrome  153–4, 204

L
late nights, occasional  184–5
leg/limb movements, NREM sleep  137
leptin  83–6, 204
lifestyle see  healthy lifestyle
light
as alertness booster  49
bedroom  182–3
blue  39–40, 47–8
dim  48
effect on mood  49–51
effects of  37–8
impact of  17
indoor / outdoor  47
influence of  51–2
internal body check  38
phase response curve  45
waking up  185
light exposure
duration and intensity  46
at night  93
regular  40–1
light perception, lack of  41
light therapy  50–1
lux  204

**M**

magnesium, blood pressure 91

mealtimes 186

melanopsin 38, 47, 204

melatonin (sleep hormone) 41–3, 47–8, 205

menopause 60–2

menstrual cycle

    effect on sleep 53, 55–7

    sleep disturbances 55–7

microsleep 205

mindfulness 194–5

mood, effect of light 49–51

mood swings/disorders, insomnia 57

motivation, lacking 111–12

movement disorders, sleep-related 129,
    136–8, 206

mPFC (medial prefrontal cortex) 115–16,
    117

muscle spasms 19

myoclonic spasms 19

**N**

naps

    afternoon 30, 33, 35, 196

    daytime 187

narcolepsy 149–52, 205

National Sleep Foundation (NSF) 27

negative thinking, causing insomnia 108,
    146–7

negativity bias 110–11, 115

neurodegenerative diseases 96

neurotransmitters 13

neutrality, losing 112–14

night terrors 158, 205

nightmares

    explained 162–3

    image rehearsal therapy (IRT) 204

    recurrent 72

noise, bedroom 183

non-24 hour sleep–wake disorder 171–2, 205

non-rapid eye movement sleep *see* NREM
    sleep

noradrenaline 117

NREM sleep 205

    alternating cycles 18

    stage 1 18–20

    stages 2 and 3 20–1

NREM-related parasomnias 156–9

**O**

obstructive sleep apnoea (OSA) 132–6

oestrogen 61

oral contraceptives 58

outdoor light 47

**P**

parasomnias

    explained 129, 155, 205

    other types 163–6

    REM-related 159–63

parasympathetic nervous system 88–9, 205

pavor nocturnes 158, 205

periodic limb movements disorder (PLMD)
    138

phase response curve 45

physical health

    quantity of sleep 81

    role of sleep 78–9

polysomnography (PSG) 205

postmenopausal women 62

postpartum period 60

'postprandial dip' 33

prefrontal cortex (PFC)

    diagram of brain 114

    effect of sleep loss 100–1

    location in brain 101

pregnancy, effect on sleep 58–60

problem-solving strategies 119–20

Process W 32

progesterone, during pregnancy 58–60

psychiatric disorders 96

    insomnia 143–4

R

racing mind
  dealing with 193–4
  not sleeping 140
rapid eye movement sleep *see* REM sleep
RBD (REM sleep behavioural disorder)
  159–60
relaxation 189–90
REM sleep
  alterations in 118–19
  alternating cycles 18
  and emotions 116–18
  explained 21–2, 205
  sleep hallucinations 151
  sleep paralysis 150–1, 160–2
REM sleep behavioural disorder (RBD)
  159–60
REM-related parasomnias 159–63
restless legs syndrome (RLS) 136–7
reward system 85
RLS (restless leg syndrome) 136–7
rotating shift workers 168
rumination
  about not sleeping 122–3, 146–7
  causing insomnia 108

S

SAD (seasonal affective disorder) 37, 50–1
SCN (suprachiasmatic nuclei) 16, 38
sexsomnia 157–8, 205
shift work disorder (SWD) 167–8
shift workers 168
short-term/transient insomnia 141
sleep
  beauty sleep 97
  best time 23–4
  boost to immune system 94–5
  effect of stress 118–23
  explained 12
  heart health 92–3
  link to diabetes 87–9
  regulation of 13–18

Slow Wave Sleep (SWS) 20–1
  what makes it happen 12–13
sleep architecture
  changes in 28
  defined 205
sleep debt 30–1, 55
sleep deprivation, study results 105–7
sleep disorders, categories 128–41
sleep drive/pressure 14, 15
sleep drunkenness 157
sleep enuresis 165, 205
sleep environment 182–4
sleep habits, healthy 22, 179–92
sleep hallucinations 164
sleep hormone (melatonin) 41–3, 47–8, 205
sleep hours, before midnight 25
sleep inertia 32–3, 206
sleep loss, most common 'form' 117
sleep maintenance insomnia 140
sleep need
  identifying 29
  personal variation 26–31
  recommended by age 27
sleep onset insomnia 140
sleep paralysis, explained 150–1, 160–2
sleep pressure/drive 195, 205
sleep sex 157–8, 205
sleep stages, dreams 68
sleep studies 54
sleep study, findings 105–7
sleep terrors 158, 205
sleepiness
  afternoon 35
  darkness and 48–9
  judging own level 105–8
  post-lunch 33–5
sleeping pills 147–8
sleep-promoting system 12–13
sleep-related breathing disorders 206
sleep-related eating disorder (SRED) 158–9
sleep-related movement disorders 206
sleeptalking 164–5

sleep–wake cycle
    desynchronized 41–2
    identifying 24–5
    managing 179
    understanding 23–4
sleepwalking 156–7
Slow Wave Sleep (SWS) 20–1
snoring 135–6
social isolation 111–12
somnambulism 156–7
somniloquy 164–5
somnipathy 206
SRED (sleep-related eating disorder) 158–9
stress
    dealing with 187
    effect on sleep 118–23
stress response 119–20
stroke, peak time 93
sunlight 185
suprachiasmatic nuclei (SCN) 16, 38
SWD (shift work disorder) 167–8
SWS (Slow Wave Sleep) 20–1
sympathetic nervous system 206
sympathovagal balance 88–9
symphony analogy 22–3

T
teenagers, DSPD 169–70
temperature, bedroom 183
threats, perception of 115–16
tiredness, signs of 197–9
travel
    minimizing jet lag 44
    westward 43–6
twitches 19
type 2 diabetes 86–90

V
vagus nerve 206
vascular tension 91

W
waking up
    healthy lifestyle 184–5
    during the night 31–2, 191
    time 55
weight gain
    appetite hormones 83–4
    hedonic drive 85
    short sleepers 82–3
'winter depression' 37, 50–1
women
    dreams 69–71
    internal body clock 54–5
    menopause 60–2
    mood swings/disorders 57
    postmenopausal 62
    restless legs syndrome 137
    sleep problems 53–4
workplace
    cognitive performance 102–3
    effect of fatigue 102–3
worry
    about not sleeping 122–3, 140, 146–7
    causing insomnia 108